Teaching Ambulatory Medicine

Teaching Ambulatory Medicine

Moving Medical Education into the Office

Samuel C. Durso, M. D.

The Johns Hopkins University Press

Baltimore and London

© 2002 The Johns Hopkins University Press
All rights reserved. Published 2002
Printed in the United States of America on acid-free paper

9 8 7 6 5 4 3 2 1

The Johns Hopkins University Press
2715 North Charles Street
Baltimore, Maryland 21218-4363
www.press.jhu.edu

Library of Congress Cataloging-in-Publication Data
Durso, Samuel C., 1954–
    Teaching ambulatory medicine : moving medical education into
the office / Samuel C. Durso.
        p. ; cm.
Includes bibliographical references and index.
    ISBN 0-8018-6903-x (pbk. : alk. paper)
    1. Ambulatory medical care—Study and teaching.
    [DNLM: 1. Ambulatory Care. 2. Education, Medical—methods.
WB 18 D966t 2002]   I. Title.
    R834 .D87 2002
    616'.0071—dc21
2001004374

A catalog record for this book is available from the British Library.

CONTENTS

Rabbi Akiva, the renowned leader of his generation, ignores the Romans' edict against teaching and is consequently arrested. A student implores his master to continue teaching him, even as his mentor sits in jail. Rabbi Akiva responds, saying, "My son, more than the calf wants to drink, the cow wants to nurse."

Talmud, Pesachim 112a

TEACHING—the act of helping someone learn—is the physician's very stock-in-trade. Nowhere is this truer than in ambulatory medicine. In this context, where most outpatient care is provided, much of the physician's work is patient education, and teaching is as crucial to the doctor's success as making a correct diagnosis or devising a workable treatment plan. For in addition to whatever medical knowledge and skill clinicians master, they must be effective communicators who grasp patients' understanding of health and use this knowledge to inform, motivate, and guide them toward goals acceptable to both. These are the essential acts of teaching and the key to the doctor's daily practice.

How much richer is this same experience when a medical student is included in patient care? For the physician committed to a life of learning, teaching the willing student in the office becomes an extension of the educator's role, and the younger colleague's inquiries become another source of professional growth and intellectual satisfaction. Let me illustrate from one of my earliest experiences with precepting in the office.

In 1981 I completed a residency in internal medicine and returned to practice in my hometown of Port Arthur, Texas. Like most newly minted internists in the 1980s, I was long on inpatient experience and short on training in ambulatory care. Removed from an academic medical center, I suddenly found myself in an inverted world—long hours in the office sandwiched between morning and afternoon rounds at the local hospital. Where before I had been accustomed to attending hospitalized patients,

I was now seeing dozens of patients a day in the office. Most were not acutely ill, but their problems were challenging just the same. The pace was dizzying. Furthermore, none of my resident clinics, whether at university, county, or Veterans Administration hospitals, resembled private practice: the patients' needs and resources were substantially different. I wondered how my previous training would be practically useful. No longer was I treating shock, adjusting ventilators, or working up fevers; instead I was dispensing advice over the telephone, counseling patients, and delegating to others care that I had once performed myself.

Office practice differed from residency in another important way. Gone were the medical students and fellow house staff. I missed their challenging questions, case discussions, and brainstorming sessions. The give-and-take of teaching and learning, I realized, had become a staple of my clinical experience. Now I was seeing patients for the most part alone, with little opportunity to share "Aha!" experiences—the small discoveries and insights that make medicine fun. This was no fault of my associates, who were as welcoming and intellectually curious as any doctors I had known. It was simply the nature of office practice: fast-paced, one patient encounter after another, with little break in between for discussing patient care.

Like most of my peers who left hospital-based training, I adapted to the requirements of ambulatory practice. Nevertheless I missed the bedside teaching that had been so much a part of residency, so I welcomed the opportunity to precept medical students in the office. This opportunity arose through the University of Texas Medical Branch in Galveston, seventy miles away. Its Department of Family Medicine was establishing a community-based residency in the city where I was practicing and needed a locally based volunteer faculty to fulfill its mission. When I inquired, the program director signed me up. In a matter of weeks I was hosting a fourth-year medical student interested in family medicine.

One of our first experiences taught me an enduring lesson about the value of ambulatory teaching. Early in the rotation, when the student was still "shadowing" me, I was covering my partner's practice while he was away. Most of the patients were new to me, and we were seeing them in quick succession. Their problems ran the gamut of ambulatory medicine, mostly minor acute illnesses and chronic disease. Inserted in the string of fifteen-minute office visits was a middle-aged woman with her aged mother in tow. I did not know the woman or her mother, and I had no chance to look through the extensive record before taking a history. The essence of the daughter's concern was that "Momma is not right." The elderly woman had no complaints and was mildly confused. The daughter was not sure how much her mother's cognitive function differed from baseline, but she insisted that "something is just not right." The older woman's temperature and blood pressure were normal, but her pulse was fast. The rest of her exam was normal except that her dress smelled like urine. Her daughter felt that any urinary incontinence was completely out of character. The medical student performed a urinalysis and discovered that the patient had a urinary tract infection. In the lab we discussed our next step. I was concerned that she might be septic. We admitted her, drew blood cultures, and administered intravenous antibiotics.

The next day her blood cultures were positive for gram-negative rods, the antibiotic coverage appeared appropriate, and the daughter confirmed that "Momma is more like herself." The student seemed impressed by his attending's "call." The hard part came next, when he asked, "What pushed you to admit her?" In the office she did not look very sick to him, and he said that he would have sent her home on oral antibiotics. I had to stop and think. My decision had been almost intuitive; now I had to explain it. Citing experience was not sufficient. I was forced to analyze my reasoning and make it understandable to him. As a result, we discussed delirium and the sometimes-subtle signs of sepsis. I could see the puzzle coming together for him. (He later told me, "I'll never forget her when I examine old patients who don't seem all that sick.") The discussion benefited me too. It solidified my own recognition of sepsis. But perhaps more important, it transformed a routine medical decision into an examined one—a process it would have been easy to skip had no student asked, "Why did you do that?" In the parlance of educators, the experience became a "teaching moment" for both of us.

After the rotation the student wrote to thank me for the experiences we shared. He said that his experience had given him a clearer appreciation of ambulatory medicine—its challenges and opportunities. I wrote back thanking him too, because on reflection I gained as much as he did. I enjoyed the camaraderie. I benefited from our mutual questions and the research they spawned. Articulating and rehearsing important concepts had enhanced my own medical knowledge. I particularly enjoyed watching him discover new ideas and gain incrementally in professional independence. And I appreciated that his need to know forced me to make medical concepts and knowledge understandable, improving my own communication with patients. Clearly, his presence contributed to my medical growth as well as to his.

Since then I have continued to teach in ambulatory settings and confirmed my original experience many times over: as much as students need and benefit from ambulatory teaching, office-based physicians benefit from providing it. It is part of our nature. We maintain and improve our skills through practice and exploration. For the physician in ambulatory practice, few exercises accomplish this more efficiently than teaching motivated learners.

The need for ambulatory teaching is undeniable. With most medical care decisions made in outpatient settings, there is strong consensus among medical educators that undergraduate and postgraduate training must include realistic ambulatory care experience (Jacobson et al. 1998). University-based preceptors can meet only a portion of the requirement, so community physicians are increasingly essential to the educational effort. I feel that physicians, whether in private practice, VA hospital ambulatory centers, HMOs, urgent care centers, free medical clinics, or public health offices, will find teaching both workable and refreshing.

Like most physicians, I have no formal training as a teacher. Nevertheless, I teach. This is what physicians do—certainly those who work effectively with patients. However, because teaching students is a special interest, I have reflected on my experience and looked for techniques that work. I have sought feedback from colleagues and gained from their experience. I have also relied on books that offer practical advice (e.g., *Precepting Medical Students in the Office,* edited by Paul M. Paulman, Jeffrey L. Susman, and Cheryl A. Abboud [Baltimore: Johns Hopkins University Press, 2000]). In the process I have improved as a teacher both for my patients and for the students who come through my office. I hope you will find these insights a helpful starting point and will find teaching in the office as enjoyable as I do.

Teaching Ambulatory Medicine

Teaching in the Office: Getting Started

Dr. Chen, who is two years out of pediatric residency, practices with a small private group in a large metropolitan area. Her growing suburban practice is approximately twenty minutes from a major medical center and draws a mix of patients with fee-for-service, HMO, and Medicaid insurance coverage. She is very happy in her work, finding it both challenging and meaningful. Now she is beginning to think about teaching in the office to share her experience with medical students and residents—but she is not sure how to start. She decides to speak to her colleagues first.

Although her partners have not seriously considered teaching medical students or residents in the office, they are not opposed to the idea. They do have questions about the effects this might have on Dr. Chen's productivity, office flow, patient satisfaction, and medical liability, among other concerns. They ask her to look into it further so they can make an informed decision.

She decides to do two things. She makes a quick literature search and finds several articles that address the questions her partners have raised about precepting and productivity, office flow, and patient satisfaction. She also contacts the pediatric residency director at the nearby medical center. Although she did not train in that program, the director is happy to meet with her and discuss her teaching interest.

The meeting goes well. The director discusses the curricular goals for ambulatory pediatric teaching and suggests that Dr. Chen attend an upcoming dinner the department holds for preceptors. The quarterly dinners are a good opportunity for community-based teachers to meet and exchange ideas. The director also arranges to have a faculty representative visit the office to meet with her and her partners and suggest ways the program can support her teaching effort. Assuming that everyone agrees, the program director will bring Dr. Chen's practice into the ambulatory teaching rotation. Based on the faculty representative's experience, she is confident that the experience will be positive for Dr. Chen, her practice, and the pediatric residents.

Dr. Jackson is an internist practicing in a semirural setting. He enjoys his work and lifestyle, but ten years into his career he is beginning to feel a little cut off from his professional colleagues. He knows that the American College of Physicians–American Society of Internal Medicine, like other primary care specialty groups, encourages members to consider office-based teaching. Indeed, its publications routinely acknowledge community-based teachers at state and national meetings. He wonders if this might be a good way to stay current and at the same time give something back to his profession. He recognizes, too, that this might increase his chance of attracting a partner in the future.

He takes a multifaceted approach to investigating his interest. He does a computer search and discovers a Web site for primary care preceptors serving rural communities. An osteopathic school administers the program. He contacts the group. He also discusses his idea with the local hospital administrator, who shares his interest in attracting new physicians to the community. The administrator thinks his hospital may contribute by providing room and board for a student. Dr. Jackson reads articles and books about office-based precepting. After several months of contacts and planning, he hosts the first student in his practice.

If you enjoy ambulatory medicine and would like to share this experience with medical students or residents, then getting started is relatively easy. With a nationwide mandate to increase ambulatory training, especially in primary care specialties such as family medicine, geriatrics, internal medicine, and pediatrics, most medical school clerkship and residency directors are eagerly looking for practicing physicians who are willing to teach medical students and postgraduates in the office. Indeed, many programs are actively recruiting community-based physicians to support this effort (Young 1996). Nevertheless, successful ambulatory teaching requires commitment from both the prospective preceptor and the affiliated training program. You must consider this and understand the potential costs in time and money. When teaching is well planned and supported, however, the physician who teaches in the office will find the experience not only practical but richly rewarding.

The first step is to confer with partners and staff.

Ambulatory teaching has a definite impact on office practice. When well organized, however, the effects are positive for students, patients, and staff alike. To bring students and residents into the practice successfully, you must build a consensus around the effort and address anticipated concerns up front.

Perhaps the most common fear staff and colleagues voice is that trainees' presence will disrupt office flow, diminish patient satisfaction, and lengthen an already long workday. In addition, they worry that teaching will cost the practice financially and reduce the preceptor's productivity. Regarding each of these concerns, staff and colleagues can be reassured. Experience confirms that ambulatory teaching, when done thoughtfully, is well accepted by patients, is easily integrated into the office flow, and need not reduce physicians' productivity.

Early on, physicians who are new to ambulatory teaching will be wise to build a little extra time into their schedules—perhaps the equivalent of one patient visit per session. This will allow additional time to supervise a student and provide patient care. However, as you might expect, experienced teachers soon learn to teach efficiently and maintain productivity (Baldwin 1997; Kearl and Mainous 1993; Usatine, Tremoulet, and Irby 2000). Also, students who are new to ambulatory medicine and those who are working in a new environment will need extra time for adjustment and orientation. But as learners gain experience this extra time becomes less important. Eventually staff will be able to schedule patients in a way (as noted in chapter 4) that permits the teacher and student to see the same number of patients together as the teacher would see alone. Students can even become assets to the practice and boost efficiency by performing procedures, reviewing records, and counseling and educating patients (Lipsky and Egan 1999). In fact, advanced students and residents who are accustomed to the teacher's practice can increase productivity by allowing the preceptor to see a few more patients per session (e.g., "walk-in" visits). In addition, as I will discuss in chapters 5, 6, and 7, there are techniques that enhance teaching efficiency. On balance the staff will learn how to create a schedule appropriate for the teacher's and learner's level of experience.

Concern about patient satisfaction should not deter physicians from teaching either students or house staff. Patients in private offices, walk-in clinics, and HMOs report satisfaction with office visits that involve teaching (Frank et al. 1997; O'Malley et al. 1997; Kirz and Larsen 1986). In fact many patients perceive greater provider interaction, enhanced education, and increased care (O'Malley et al. 1997). Though it may be surprising, patients rarely mind repeating parts of the examination, discussing personal matters, or extending the office visit as a result of teaching students (Devera-Sales, Paden, and Vinson 1999). Staff can promote a positive perception of office-based teaching by taking part and by their own enthusiasm for the mission. And of course patients who do not have the time or inclination to be seen by a learner are always given the choice to see the preceptor alone.

The time spent teaching should not have a major impact on the duration of the staff's workday if the teacher works efficiently. Most of the time spent with students and residents—averaging three hours per half-day session—is concurrent with patient care. Indeed, this one-to-one contact is the primary value of office-based teaching. Additional time spent alone with the student, approximately an hour a day, usually occurs during breaks or at the end of the day. This should not require the staff to stay longer than usual. Although time spent with the learner usually lengthens the teacher's day, most find the professional companionship and discussions well worth the effort (Vinson et al. 1997). When problems with patient flow or overruns do occur, remedies such as those outlined in chapter 7 nearly always work.

Colleagues might wonder as well if medical students and house staff increase patient care costs, as sometimes occurs on inpatient services. Office-based teaching, however, does not seem to increase patient costs through additional lab work, prescriptions, or referrals (Frank et al. 1977), since management decisions are ultimately the supervising physician's. Partners should know, too, that liability coverage for students and house staff is borne by their training institutions.

What does ambulatory teaching cost a typical practice? Experiences vary, but many physicians report no increased cost (Vinson and Paden 1994). As I noted above, some physicians may see one patient fewer per session, usually with novice learners (Kirz and Larsen 1986; Osborn, Sargent, and Williams 1993). If that same physician sees a few more patients per session with more experienced students, then the loss is balanced by the gain. This often happens as a student or resident gains experience over the course of a rotation. However, there may be other ways to realize partial financial compensation. Some training programs provide a small stipend to the preceptor. Recently schools have negotiated small capitation increases for affiliated teaching practices (Grayson et al. 1999). Even benefits such as tuition for continuing education courses, continuing education credits for teaching (category 2 CME), library access, e-mail, Internet service, and books, though small monetarily, are appreciable (Alguire et al. 2001). In the end most teachers observe that the greatest benefits are not monetary but rather come from the increased energy that eager learners bring to the office (Fulkerson and Wang-Cheng 1997). Once teaching is up and running, preceptors and their staffs and colleagues will likely share in the satisfaction that comes with contributing to their profession.

If teaching in the office looks promising, then the next step is contacting the appropriate school or training program and exploring a mutually agreeable teaching arrangement.

Area alumni are a good resource for schools and teaching programs that are reaching out to their communities. Of course you need not be a graduate of a nearby medical or osteopathic school or residency training program to call the educational office, department head, or program director for your specialty. Remember, too, that primary care programs in one specialty—say internal medicine—are often happy to place students with those in an allied specialty such as family medicine. Both the Association of American Medical Colleges (AAMC) and the American Association of Colleges of Osteopathic Medicine maintain listings of medical and osteopathic colleges in the United States. Web links to individual schools through the AAMC site are very helpful for locating participating medical schools. Specific contact information can easily be obtained from these sites. Also, the American Medical Student Association maintains a Web-accessible list of student community rotations.

Association of American Medical Colleges
2450 N Street, NW
Washington, DC 20037-1126
(202) 828-0400
http://www.aamc.org

American Association of Colleges of Osteopathic Medicine
5550 Friendship Boulevard, Suite 300
Chevy Chase, MD 20815-7201
(301) 968-4100
http://www.aacom.org

American Medical Student Association
1902 Association Drive
Reston, VA 20191-9831
(800) 767-2266
http://www.amsa.org

Colleagues who already participate in ambulatory teaching can make sound recommendations. They can also supply referrals for programs looking for community-based teachers, and they should be able to introduce interested physicians to their teaching program directors. Also, their experience in getting started is valuable. Potential community-based preceptors can also contact faculty responsible for ambulatory teaching through their local, state, or national medical organizations.

Some physicians who are interested in office-based teaching get their start by helping to teach physical diagnosis to second-year medical students. Besides building your skills and reputation as a teacher, this rewarding experience (for which preceptors are always in demand) helps forge contact with faculty members who are likely to know a training program's needs. In addition, these very students may later choose rotations or electives in the preceptor's office. Similarly, physicians who volunteer in free medical clinics may find house staff eager to work alongside them. This opportunity builds experience in precepting and is a viable way to begin ambulatory teaching.

Physicians who are far from regional training centers may find starting and sustaining ambulatory teaching a little more involved (e.g., travel, housing), but schools increasingly are working to make this succeed. Area Health Education Centers funded through the U.S. Department of Health and Human Services can assist. Individual health education centers can easily be found by typing "area health education center" into most search engines. In addition to these suggestions, national and state medical societies and specialty groups can help practitioners make contact with interested medical and osteopathic schools. The Web sites for the American Academy of Family Physicians, the Society of Teachers of Family Medicine, the American College of Physicians–American Society of Internal Medicine, and the American Academy of Pediatrics are particularly helpful for identifying opportunities for preceptors, links to preceptor groups, and information about office-based teaching.

American Academy of Family Physicians
11400 Tomahawk Creek Parkway, Suite 540
Leawood, KS 66211
(800) 274-2237
http://www.aafp.org

Society of Teachers of Family Medicine
11400 Tomahawk Creek Parkway, Suite 540
Leawood, KS 66211
(800) 274-2237
http://www.stfm.org

American College of Physicians–American Society
    of Internal Medicine
190 North Independence Mall West
Philadelphia, PA 19106-1572
(800) 523-1546
http://www.acponline.org

Area Health Education Center
Department of Health and Human Services
Division of Medicine, Room 9A27
Parklawn Building
5600 Fishers Lane
Rockville, MD 20857
(301) 443-6950

Finally, beyond your own commitment to teach, it is important to have
the support of a preceptor program (DeWitt, Goldberg, and Roberts 1993;
DeWitt 1996). Of course the extent of this support will depend on your responsibilities. If possible, it is ideal to have a training program representative visit the practice site. During that visit the preceptor can get a clear
picture of the curricular goals, discuss stipends and other support, including faculty development, and work out how to address problems should
they occur. Even if a site visit is not practical, these same issues will need
to be discussed.

Ultimately the decision to teach medical students or residents in the office requires careful consideration, since precepting definitely has costs in time and energy, if not always money. However, the rewards are many, including increased learning and a renewed joy in practicing ambulatory medicine. With planning and support, physicians who invite students or residents into their offices will almost certainly enjoy success.

Summary

- Primary care and other specialties recognize the need, and indeed the mandate, to increase opportunities for their trainees to practice in a variety of ambulatory settings.
- Physicians interested in sharing their professional skills with medical students and residents will have little trouble finding medical schools and other postgraduate training programs willing to support office-based teaching.
- Teaching in a wide variety of ambulatory settings is not only possible but also highly satisfying—yet it entails costs. The prospective teacher must consider this when planning to implement teaching in the office.
- The first step is to understand and anticipate the effects teaching may have on office flow, patient satisfaction, and physician productivity.
- Ambulatory teaching experience in many settings has shown that teaching is compatible with workable office flow, that patients are remarkably satisfied with care that involves teaching, and that physicians can both teach and maintain realistic productivity. Furthermore, most teaching programs support community-based teachers with stipends or other tangible benefits.
- Practitioners in both metropolitan and rural locations will discover that schools and residencies are reaching out to community physicians. Initial contact therefore is relatively easy to make.
- In addition to the educational departments of nearby schools, local, regional, and national organizations can be of great assistance in helping physicians locate and approach an appropriate training program.
- Much information supporting ambulatory precepting is available through the Internet.

2

The Goals of Teaching Medicine in the Ambulatory Setting

A senior medical student examines a mother and daughter in a community-based family medicine clinic. Both appear to have a scabies infestation, and the medical student identifies what looks to be a half-centimeter linear burrow on the child's hand. Unsure of her next step, she excuses herself briefly from the examining room and describes the finding to the medical director. After confirming the student's finding, he walks her through the procedure of uncovering the burrow and preparing a covered slide. Ten minutes later the two make a positive diagnosis when they identify a scabies mite under the microscope.

An internist stands unobtrusively to the side while a medical student takes a history from a middle-aged man who has been suffering from chronic headaches. Before he begins to examine the patient, the medical student asks the senior physician if there are any additional questions he would ask the patient. The doctor acknowledges the thoroughness of the student's history to this point, noting that he now has a good description of the headache's location, duration, character, and mitigating factors, but he wonders if the patient has any deeper concern, aside from the pain, that has caused him to seek medical attention. The man hesitates briefly, then says that a year ago his wife's brother died of brain cancer. Later the medical student and physician discuss nonverbal clues to patients' stress and the unspoken reasons behind many outpatient visits.

A female pediatric resident spends several afternoons a week with a pediatrician who is also a working mother. Over a short time the two develop a strong respect for each other's ability. The resident especially enjoys the informal time they spend together over lunch. She appreciates it when the senior colleague shares her experience in balancing family and work, something she often wonders about.

Consider the three vignettes above. They portray different, but valid, roles for the clinician-teacher. To be sure, she is a repository of knowledge and experience. But she also must be a capable communicator who transmits medical knowledge and patient care skills effectively. Furthermore, the teacher is a shaper and role model who recognizes students' needs and guides their professional development as well as an adviser and mentor who listens and willingly shares time with a junior colleague. The experienced clinician provides a seasoned perspective and perhaps encouragement, all while caring for patients in the ambulatory care setting.

Clearly then, office-based teaching is a complex task, and caring for a patient in a student's presence is not the same as teaching ambulatory medicine; if it were, then passive observation would suffice and the student could be content to watch the physician go about the daily routine. Rather, teaching is active (and interactive). Like patient care, it is a collaboration involving dialogue and understanding between two parties (Schwenk and Whitman 1987). To teach effectively the physician must use discernment, engagement, and feedback—all the skills necessary for the patient's education—to the student's benefit. Furthermore, much of the content of medicine—the actual practice and professional conduct—can be learned only by doing. Therefore teachers must involve students and be involved with them in both clinical and professional matters. Dry lectures and reading assignments will not do. To be involved the teacher must assess the learner's needs, develop goals that are compatible with the student's professional growth, and negotiate a plan to achieve these. In other words, the prospective teacher must know what to expect from the learner and understand what the learner expects from the teacher.

Broadly speaking then, what are the goals of teaching medicine in the ambulatory setting?

While many teaching goals and objectives are specific and depend on the course curriculum and particular students' needs, the general intent of teaching ambulatory medicine is to impart professional knowledge, skills, and values used by physicians in the setting where most patient care decisions are made. These can be characterized as *educational goals* and *educational objectives*. In addition to this, most students want something less tangible, but also important—a glimpse of their possible future. This is often an unstated goal of the ambulatory teaching mission. It includes the chance to exercise some autonomy while knowing a supervisor is close by.

It includes practicing medicine in the "real world" where the student gets the feel of a doctor's day. It even includes seeing the doctor interact with family, friends, and colleagues and act as a citizen within the larger society.

Thus the teacher's aim is to help the learner acquire patient care skills and share a professional experience. Some goals and objectives are explicit; these can be oral or written (e.g., curricular, learning contract). Some remain unarticulated and are simply implicit in the teacher's and learner's experience together. Much of this depends on the pair's judgment and the fluid nature of ambulatory practice.

Educational Goals

Once a teacher identifies a learner's needs, effective teaching begins with establishing clear educational goals. Teaching without goals is like a journey without a destination. A traveler who has no clear destination might experience pleasant surprises and memorable highlights along the way but also risks wasting time and missing opportunities.

Goals, broadly speaking, are defined as the end toward which the educational effort is directed (Kern et al. 1998). More specifically, the term *educational goal* is used to indicate an overarching statement of educational intent, and an *educational objective* denotes a measurable outcome that supports the student's attainment of that goal. Measurable outcomes can take various forms: demonstrating knowledge (e.g., passing a test, answering the preceptor's questions, delivering a talk, solving a problem); performing a specific task (e.g., demonstrating a skill); or spending a specified time doing something (e.g., participating in a discussion or attending a clinic). Objectives specify who will do what, and when. In each instance the teacher determines whether the student has acquired the desired information, skill, or exposure.

For example, an educational goal for medical students in ambulatory pediatrics might be to demonstrate proficiency in performing well-baby examinations. This is rather general, but it provides a direction for the teacher and student. Knowing the goal leads to developing objectives that measure the student's achievement. An educational objective that supports proficiency in well-baby exams, for instance, might entail satisfactorily recording and interpreting behavioral milestones during five well-baby visits under a preceptor's supervision. Thus the goals are broad and may encompass several objectives; objectives are specific and provide yardsticks for measuring achievement. The goal does not specify concrete opportunities for the teacher to assess the student. The objective presents a specific task, and the attending uses it to determine how well the student meets that milestone.

Major goals should be made explicit. Usually the course director guides students to choose significant and attainable goals. These may be oral or written, though written goals are preferable. In either case they can be formulated into an agreement between teacher and student. The agreement specifies how goals and objectives will be taught and forms the basis of a *learning contract* (see chapter 5). The learning contract is negotiated and agreed on at the beginning of a rotation. It may be renegotiated and modified along the way. This agreement provides clear targets for teacher and learner and helps the teacher organize clinical experiences that meet these targets. Goals and objectives that are stated and agreed on are more likely to be fulfilled. There is less chance that either party will misunderstand his responsibility or become disappointed by unmet expectations. Furthermore, explicit goals and objectives make it easier for teacher and student to determine each other's progress toward educational end points. The teacher can review these with the student and, if necessary, decide what adjustments are necessary—whether this entails altering the teaching method, case mix, use of time, or other aspects.

A curriculum committee often determines major goals and objectives for core ambulatory rotations in internal medicine, family medicine, and pediatrics. Schools want their graduates to achieve specific competencies and therefore specify these for rotations typically lasting a month to six weeks. When schools design a well-written curriculum that includes goals and objectives, these become the foundation for a working contract between teacher and learner. Some programs may not have done so, and in that case the teacher should take responsibility for developing goals and objectives with the student.

Even when goals are determined by the curriculum, the teacher and student can modify them or set new goals if needed. This may arise out of an ongoing assessment and dialogue with the student—for instance, new educational needs may become apparent or circumstances may change during the rotation. Consider the following examples: the patient mix does not meet the student's needs, the schedule changes, teaching opportunities with other providers become available, the student discovers a new interest and wants to pursue it, or the teacher identifies a previously unrecognized deficiency in a student's knowledge. When this occurs, a change in course necessitates developing new goals and objectives. The basis for this flexibility is the teacher's judgment and a willingness to accept the student as a collaborator. Obviously it may be wise to discuss significant changes in educational goals with course directors, but reasonable latitude in formulating educational goals is to be expected when, in the teacher's judgment, a change furthers the student's development.

Of course, much teaching that occurs during an ambulatory rotation is neither planned nor part of the predetermined curriculum—impromptu teaching moments and student-initiated electives come to mind. Even during an ambulatory rotation for which definite goals have been set, important teaching points will arise that are not encompassed by general goals or specific objectives. For example, a student who intends to learn skin biopsy methods from a dermatologist may also learn how to obtain informed consent even though this was not a specific learning objective. Nevertheless, goals that are written or communicated orally clarify the purpose and help the teacher meet the student's primary needs. Articulated goals will not prevent the teacher and student from using unplanned teaching opportunities to learn additional skills.

Most explicit goals in ambulatory teaching, whether derived from a course curriculum or from the student's personal interest, are based on the student's need to acquire clinical skills. (Exceptions are goals that may not be explicit, such as the opportunity to discuss career choices, and they will be discussed later.) Clinical skills are often classified in one of the following domains: cognitive, psychomotor, or affective (Bloom 1956; Harrow 1972; Krathwohl, Bloom, and Masia 1980).

Cognitive Skills

Cognitive skills demonstrate knowing and thinking. They include the ability to perceive, remember, understand, make judgments, and solve problems. Basic functions such as knowing and remembering are sometimes referred to as "lower-order" skills in contrast to "higher-order" thinking that requires more complex intellectual functions such as forming judgments and solving problems. Lower-order skills are easier to teach and measure because the student can list, cite, or identify the information requested. Higher-order thinking skills such as reasoning, judgment, or problem solving are harder to teach and measure, since doing so requires testing the student's thinking processes, usually with probing questions.

Psychomotor Skills

Psychomotor skills require mental acumen to perform nontrivial motor or sensory tasks. In this domain, movement, sight, speech, hearing, and touch are used in the service of such diverse tasks as physical examination, history taking, communicating with patients, and performing diagnostic and other procedural skills. "Performing" and "doing" characterize psychomotor skills.

Affective Skills

Affective skills (sometimes referred to as attitudinal skills) derive from the learner's values, beliefs, reactions, and emotions, and physicians use them to interpret and respond to patients' cognitive, behavioral, psychological, and spiritual needs. Verbal and nonverbal skills (e.g., "healing touch," facial expression, eye contact, voice tone) are often needed to interpret affective information and transmit it to patients. This domain must often be inferred from the student's behavior.

Naturally, the clinician uses all these skills concurrently when caring for a patient. In most instances they are so interwoven into the clinical encounter that the physician would consider them inseparable. Yet it is helpful to view them separately to help the teacher observe and analyze the student's clinical skills. The following example illustrates cognitive, psychomotor, and affective skills as they might be used in the evaluation and management of a common clinical problem.

A student examines a middle-aged male with an acutely painful hot and swollen knee. As part of the evaluation and management of this patient, the student must recognize the problem, categorize it as an example of acute monoarticular arthritis, develop a differential diagnosis, understand the diagnostic and therapeutic options, and make appropriate choices (cognitive skills: know, recognize, reason, judge). He takes a history and examines the patient. He then aspirates the joint and examines the fluid with a microscope (psychomotor skills: do, perform). He anticipates and responds to the patient's fear of pain, values the patient as an autonomous decision maker, and negotiates a treatment that is acceptable to the patient (affective skills: empathize, value).

Goals and objectives can be developed that reflect skills in each of these clinical domains. Categorizing skills in this way helps the teacher to develop goals and objectives that encompass appropriate competencies and to monitor progress in each of the domains for any given clinical encounter.

For example, consider a curriculum designed to promote proficiency in preventive health care. It might state the following general goals:

1. The student will understand the principles and accepted practice of primary and secondary preventive health care (cognitive).

2. During routine ambulatory office visits the student will discuss with patients and perform appropriate primary and secondary preventive care (psychomotor).

3. The student will respect patients' right to accept or refuse preventive health care recommendations (affective).

Specific objectives are developed that are then used to demonstrate mastery of each of these goals. If a student needs to develop competency in preventive health care, the course directors might decide that performing specific tasks is appropriate to confirm the achievement of these goals. In this case the teacher identifies the following objectives and uses these to evaluate the student's skill in screening and managing hypertension:

1. The student will be able to define normal and high-normal blood pressure and mild, moderate, and severe hypertension (cognitive).

2. The student will demonstrate the correct technique for measuring blood pressure (psychomotor).

3. The student will understand the patient's perception of hypertension and consider the patient's treatment preferences when devising a comprehensive preventive health strategy (affective).

In this example goals and objectives were chosen to illustrate skills in each domain. Goals and objectives may be exclusively in one domain, in more than one, or in all three depending on the educational need. Illustrations are provided in table 2.1.

By identifying goals and objectives and considering their domains, the teacher and student can accomplish the following:

• Choose the appropriate content during a learning experience (e.g., facts, skills, and values)
• Use an optimal teaching method (e.g., lectures, practice, modeling) to achieve these goals
• Define the teacher's and student's responsibilities (e.g., the teacher will watch the student perform a patient interview and provide feedback immediately after the session; the student will perform the following activities—when, where, and how often)
• Organize teaching resources (e.g., case mix, references, visual-aid equipment or other educational material, location of teaching, etc.)
• Set priorities to emphasize the most important teaching points
• Avoid missing goals and neglecting domains
• Monitor the student's progress and provide feedback
• Measure achievement
• Define new goals that had not been identified earlier

This illustration demonstrates how a clinician can use knowledge of the student's goals and the skill domains to evaluate and respond to a teaching opportunity.

An internist meets a medical student at the beginning of an ambulatory medicine rotation to review goals. They discuss the student's educational experience and current needs. Both agree on goals that follow from the course curriculum and the student's interests. One goal is to understand and incorporate age-appropriate preventive health measures into routine office visits.

During the rotation the preceptor takes an opportunity to supervise as the student performs routine preventive care for an overweight young woman. She watches the student use a blood pressure cuff and mercury manometer, observing her interaction with the patient and the technique she uses to measure the pa-

tient's blood pressure. Immediately after the visit, the attending discusses the significance of the visit and findings with the student.

Before this encounter the teacher anticipates many potential lessons, but she chooses to focus on some and not others. Which ones? Having reviewed the student's educational goals, she is able to ask the following questions:

• What are the educational goals and objectives (cognitive, psychomotor, or affective) contracted with the student? How can I use this clinical encounter to help her achieve them? For instance, does the student have a goal that is specifically suited to this visit, such as accurately measuring the blood pressure (psychomotor skills)? Or are there perhaps other goals, not unique to this patient visit but just as important, such as establishing rapport and putting the patient at ease (affective skills)?

• Looked at another way, what elements of this patient-student interaction require cognitive, psychomotor, or affective skills, and what is the best method for teaching any one of them? For instance, can the student effectively use the information she obtains from measuring the blood pressure? Would she benefit from a focused talk or from reading about the ambulatory evaluation and management of hypertension (cognitive domain)? Did she use acceptable technique to measure the patient's blood pressure? (Did she select a cuff size appropriate to the patient's arm circumference?) If not, the preceptor might demonstrate this skill or, better yet, have the student perform the measurements with the teacher's guidance (psychomotor domain).

• Are skills in one or more domains being emphasized to the exclusion of others? For example, is too little emphasis being placed on affective skills? Perhaps the teacher is focusing exclusively on factual knowledge or psychomotor skills while missing opportunities to teach important affective skills. The teacher who is concerned about developing the student's professional attitude about patient care might consider increased observation, feedback, and modeling of specific behavior. Perhaps she will prompt the student to ask the patient about her perceived health (e.g., How will a diagnosis of hypertension likely affect the patient's

Table 2.1. Goals and Objectives

Goals	Objectives
Knowledge domain (actions: knows, understands, defines, reasons, solves, and judges)	
Student will recognize, diagnose, and cost-effectively treat the most common medical problems in adult ambulatory practice.	1. List the most common diseases in ambulatory practice and compare with patient log completed at the end of the rotation.
	2. Demonstrate competence to diagnose and treat most common problems.
	3. Estimate and defend the cost of therapy for five patients treated by the student.
Student will understand the purpose of advance directives. Student will recognize situations for which advance directives are most appropriate.	1. Student will define competency, coma, vegetative state, terminal illness, health care agent, durable power of attorney, and living will.
	2. Student will complete Web-based module end-of life ethical dilemmas.
	3. During rotation, student will identify five patients for whom it is appropriate to discuss advance directives and discuss with the preceptor.
Student will know the most common causes of back pain and be able to distinguish dangerous from benign causes.	1. Student will spend one session a week in back clinic with an orthopedic specialist.
	2. Student will present one case of back pain in conference each week.
	3. Student will read chapter on back pain and deliver short talk on causes and evidence-based treatment of back pain.
Psychomotor skills (actions: does, performs, demonstrates, and shows)	
Student will be able to perform comprehensive and focused histories and physical exams.	1. Attending will observe and provide feedback on one comprehensive and one focused exam performed by the student each week.
	2. By the end of the rotation, student will be able to elicit the patient's chief concern,

Table 2.1. (continued)

Goals	Objectives
	making appropriate use of open and closed questions.
	3. By the final week of the rotation, student will demonstrate competency examining each of the major organ systems specified in the curriculum.
Resident will demonstrate skill evaluating and managing problems by telephone.	1. Resident will spend two sessions working with the triage nurse taking patients' telephone calls.
	2. Resident will document telephone advice in patients' records.

Affective or attitudinal skills (actions: feelings, values, reactions, and convictions)

Student will demonstrate respect for cultural values when making treatment recommendations.	1. Student will participate in a group discussion focusing on cultural values and their effect on treatment choices.
	2. Student and attending will identify their own values (specified) and discuss how these might help or hinder their patient care.
Student will work collaboratively with office staff to appreciate their contribution to patient care.	1. Student will work with the receptionist, billing clerk, and medical records clerk one half-day session each during the rotation.
	2. Student will follow one patient through the check-in and check-out process.
	3. Student will attend monthly office staff meeting and discuss the experience with the preceptor.

perception of well-being?), thus helping her gain insight from a real-life experience. Alternatively, she could use the experience with this patient as a case discussion and develop the idea more deeply later.

• Is the student meeting her major goals and demonstrating competency in the course objectives? Perhaps adjustments need to be made in the schedule, the case mix, or teaching techniques in order to accomplish these objectives.

• Has the teacher reviewed goals and objectives with the student during evaluation sessions?

• Has the teacher provided and received feedback to determine how well the two are achieving the purpose of teaching?

• Is there an opportunity to teach a point that was not an explicit educational goal or objective? Perhaps the teacher recognizes a teaching moment that should not be overlooked. For instance, she notices a highly desirable behavior and wants to reinforce it (e.g., when the student uses understandable, nontechnical language to communicate with patients) even though it is not an explicit goal or objective. Alternatively, perhaps a deficiency in the student's interviewing skill becomes apparent and the teacher wants to correct the problem while the experience is fresh (e.g., the student interrupts the patient's answers).

• Based on the teacher's observation, should the two consider adding new goals and objectives to the learning contract?

Of course the preceptor need not ask all these questions before every teaching encounter. Some of this exercise, understandably, is set aside for later reflection or made part of an ongoing review of the teaching experience. Still, the example shows that an ordinary clinical encounter produces a wealth of teaching opportunities. Consequently, many lessons could be derived from any one teaching encounter. The sheer volume of teaching points could become overwhelming were the teacher not able to keep an eye on the goals and objectives. Remembering them helps in organizing the learner's needs and setting priorities. The teacher and student should determine these goals and objectives at the beginning of a rotation and review them periodically to ensure that the teaching endeavor is achieving its purpose.

Regarding learning goals in the cognitive, psychomotor, and affective domains, two points should be made. One, when teaching there is a tendency to emphasize cognitive and psychomotor skills while neglecting affective skills. Two, cognitive and psychomotor skills are easier to measure than affective skills, in part because it is easier to develop objectives for cognitive and psychomotor skills (e.g., list the causes for monoarticular arthritis, demonstrate the proper technique for joint aspiration) than for affective skills (e.g., demonstrate respect for patients' modesty during physical exams). Nevertheless, these points only highlight the utility of making goals and objectives explicit and considering the domains they represent. By doing this and monitoring the student's progress toward achieving them, the teacher avoids neglecting skills in one or more domains. Also, although outcomes for affective skills are less easily measured, this does not diminish the value of setting clear objectives in this domain if this is a teaching priority. Setting goals simply provides a recognizable target.

Some educators make the point that many useful teaching goals fall outside the parameters of a curriculum and cannot be easily measured (Anderson and Faust 1973). Teaching opportunities will arise, for instance, that are not encompassed by existing goals. Some of these may be called teaching moments—memorable experiences that impart valuable lessons. Furthermore, as I noted in the beginning, there are benefits to the student-teacher relationship, such as modeling professional behavior, that are hard to quantify. Finally, self-directed learners will freely create new goals and modify old ones when this makes sense. There must be room for creativity where the unexpected teaching opportunity occurs. Having too many explicit goals risks overwhelming and distracting the teaching process, and the teacher and student will feel burdened trying to make every encounter conform to a script or checklist. Therefore it is important that goals be reasonable in number and achievable. Neither the teacher nor the student should feel permanently bound to a master plan that limits revision or renegotiation of learning targets. The point, simply, is that predetermined goals, to the extent that they are helpful, serve as guideposts. With goals in mind, the teacher and student work more efficiently.

Indirect Benefits of Teaching Ambulatory Medicine

What about the many benefits of teaching that are incidental to the explicit educational goals? Certainly there is a great purpose to pairing students with experienced physicians in addition to imparting knowledge and skills (Jaffe, Friedman, and Ritchen 1985). What experiences can the teacher and student expect beyond the learning contract? There are many valuable by-products of the experience:

- Developing a positive collegial relationship
- Discussing professional goals
- Professional role modeling
- Observing the doctor-patient relationship
- Recruitment to primary care and geriatric medicine
- Enhanced practice prestige
- Continued learning by the teacher
- Teaching the learner to teach

Developing a Positive Collegial Relationship

Medical training is often stressful. Working in a supportive environment with a single mentor is a welcome respite for many medical students and postgraduates in training. Also, students are afraid of not knowing and fear the consequences this may have for their patients. Expressing these feelings to a supportive mentor is reassuring. There are precious few opportunities for students and residents to have lengthy, uninterrupted time with a mentor on inpatient services. This is one of the few opportunities during training where the learner has the support and encouragement of an experienced preceptor. Finally, there is the comradeship the teacher enjoys. Having a student share your excitement about medicine is professionally energizing. Clinicians who volunteer to teach do so in part because they enjoy building relationships—and learners naturally appreciate and respond to this.

Discussing Professional Goals

Pressure to make career decisions begins early in medical school and residency. It is not uncommon for students, residents, and even fellows—whose careers appear to be on a well-marked path—to want time with a mentor whose experience they value. Unfortunately, mentors with time are hard to find. The ambulatory practice, though frequently busy, is more accommodating in this regard, with informal opportunities for discussion over lunch, after hours, and the like. Even if their careers are different from one the student is considering, older colleagues can offer wise coun-

sel. The experience they have gained while making career decisions is valuable in its own right.

Professional Role Modeling

Medicine is by tradition a way of life demanding responsibility to yourself, family, patients, colleagues, and society (Swick 2000). In addition to
clinical skills, the successful professional adopts values such as generosity,
empathy, caring, patience, equanimity, and thoroughness. These cannot
be taught didactically; they are best learned by emulation. Furthermore,
physicians must learn to balance professional and personal life, which requires forethought and reflection. Spending time with a clinician who
models this balance is an invaluable experience. Students need opportunities to discuss these aspects of medical life, and ambulatory rotations are
well suited for this.

Observing the Doctor-Patient Relationship

In recent decades the doctor-patient relationship has evolved from an authoritarian model to a collaborative one. In other words, physicians know
that top-down instructions to patients are often ineffective. Consultation
and persuasion that consider the patient's values and goals are often more
effective than "doctor's orders." Collaborative decisions between the doctor and patient are therefore ideal and are most likely to be evident in an
outpatient setting. Unlike hospitalized patients, who are sick and dependent on others for care and decisions, ambulatory patients are usually in a
better position to exercise autonomy in their medical decisions. Furthermore, the medical office is the setting where most counseling, patient education, and negotiation occur. Students are apt to see patients who are
actively making decisions in an entirely different light than they experience on inpatient services. The ambulatory practice gives students and
postgraduates more time to see senior doctors conversing with their patients than is typical during hospital rounds. Also, the student sees the
doctor-patient relationship develop over an extended period, again uncommon in other settings.

Recruitment to Primary Care and Geriatric Medicine

Except for medical schools and postgraduate programs specifically designed to recruit primary care physicians, most medical students and res-

idents see role models in the hospital long before they work with physicians in the office. Thus they have little exposure to primary care practice
early in their careers. Furthermore, hospital-based ambulatory clinics
offer only limited exposure to primary care. The varieties of experience
available in private offices, managed care systems, and urgent care centers
differ from those in academic ambulatory care environments and are important for creating a comprehensive medical education. This is true for
both pediatrics and adult medicine, including geriatrics (Lavizzo-Mourey
et al. 1990; Burke et al. 1995). Until students or residents encounter the
challenge of evaluating and managing medical illness outside the hospital's bulwark of technology, with a more varied patient base, they will not
appreciate just how demanding and satisfying primary care is. Some will
decide this is the kind of medical career they want to pursue.

Enhanced Practice Prestige

Patients and colleagues justifiably respect good teachers. Effective teaching is evidence of professional mastery, and clinicians who teach are recognized for their love of learning. Patients frequently express pride in
having physicians whom others trust to pass along their expertise. Furthermore, the exercise of teaching in patients' presence reveals to them
just how much thought goes into medical reasoning and often builds their
confidence in their medical care.

Continued Learning by the Teacher

Teaching has many rewards, none more satisfying than continuing to
learn. The sources are preparation for teaching and the students themselves, who bring not only questions worth exploring but knowledge from
centers where ideas are continually being generated. Teaching forces you
to develop expertise. You cannot teach without mastering a concept and
repeating it to each new cohort of students. Also, meeting a student's educational needs forces critical appraisal of your own knowledge. "Am I
right?" becomes the touchstone before every statement the teacher makes.

Teaching the Learner to Teach

As I noted before, teaching is what doctors do. It is a skill necessary both
for patient care and for communicating with colleagues. Many future
teachers will practice what they have seen. If the ambulatory clinician

provides a good model, students should learn valuable lessons that improve patient care and communicative skills. One hopes, too, that some of these students will accept the challenge to pass along their knowledge to a new generation of professionals.

Summary

- The ambulatory setting is a rich venue for teaching.
- Opportunities for the clinician to teach ambulatory medicine are abundant in most communities.
- Teaching skills flow directly from many of the analytical and patient education skills that clinicians already use.
- Teaching begins with understanding the educational goals of the learner.
- Educational goals can be divided into cognitive, psychomotor, and affective domains.
- Using these, the teacher can analyze a clinical encounter in light of students' needs and help them achieve their learning goals.
- Finally, ambulatory teaching provides many valuable indirect benefits. These include developing a collegial relationship with a mentor, finding time to discuss professional goals, professional role modeling, observing the doctor-patient relationship, recruitment to primary care and geriatrics, enhanced practice prestige, continued learning by the teacher, and teaching the learner to teach.

3

Adult Learning

Helping Adults Learn

Having completed basic sciences, two third-year medical students begin clinical medicine. Part of the tract includes a longitudinal ambulatory care experience with a family medicine group. Besides supervised patient care, the weekly sessions include case-based didactic lectures and round table discussions concerning such topics as the doctor-patient relationship and professional values. The students seem comfortable in the didactic sessions and take notes assiduously, but they feel anxious because the round table sessions lack defined content. They are more comfortable when given explicit principles or facts. They seem reluctant to enter the group discussions. This reticence is overcome, however, when each prepares a challenging patient encounter for discussion. By the end of the rotation they appreciate how much they have learned from the directed exchange. Furthermore, they can articulate new insights that have shaped their interactions with patients.

A student nurse-practitioner intends to concentrate on women's health after graduation. She uses an elective month to work with a gynecologist in community practice. Her primary goal is to strengthen her skill at performing pelvic exams and Pap smears. At the beginning of the rotation the gynecologist gives her a handout that describes Pap smear technique, suggests focused reading, and works with her using an anatomical model. Later, as she is becoming proficient, he suggests she make arrangements with the hospital pathologist to "follow" her Pap smear slides from the office through the pathology department. In this way she will learn first-hand how her technique affects slide quality and results.

An internal medicine fellow is interested in how health policy affects the elderly. To gain more ambulatory clinical experience with the problems of older patients, he visits a geriatrician's office once a week for a year. A healthy seventy-eight-year-old woman asks his advice about breast cancer screening. Although he knows the adult cancer screening guidelines and Medicare coverage for mammography, he realizes he does not know the absolute risks and benefits of breast cancer screening for women over age seventy, nor does he know how to incorporate information about comorbidity into his recommendation. He determines that he will need to research this question before he can answer her. The geriatrician serves as his adviser and resource.

As I noted in chapter 1, clinicians practicing ambulatory medicine rely on teaching skills every day—usually as part of patient education. They know that adults bring varying backgrounds, learning styles, knowledge, and skills to learning. Furthermore, they know from their own experience that much professional learning is self-directed and motivated by a perceived need to know. Therefore even a preceptor who has never studied adult education will recognize many of the following principles that promote adult learning (Darkenwald and Merriam 1982; Knowles 1973; Ericksen 1985).

1. Learning is enhanced by preparation, previous learning, and experience.

2. Learning that is self-motivated is likely to be eagerly pursued and durable.

3. Feedback, knowledge of results, and positive reinforcement promote learning.

4. Information presented in an organized form is more easily learned.

5. Repetition improves retention.

6. Tasks that are meaningful and applicable are learned more easily.

7. Active participation improves learning.

8. A supportive but challenging environment nurtures learning.

Preparation

Learners need prerequisite skills and knowledge before beginning to work toward a new objective (Anderson and Faust 1973). Acquired skills and knowledge provide the structure on which students organize new facts, and the continuity of new knowledge in a sequence with previous knowledge enhances recall. The teacher may make assumptions about the learner's knowledge based on experience. In many cases a quick test, such as asking questions, is sufficient to ensure that the level of instruction is not below or above the student's ability. When necessary the teacher prepares the student with the basic information, materials, and orientation to promote learning.

Intrinsic Motivation

Motivation, in this context, means a desire to know. A student who perceives something as worth knowing will pursue it, but teaching that is imposed will not enjoy the same success. In general students and postgraduates on ambulatory rotations have a high desire to learn, and they value clinical skills. Even when clinical skills do not appear valuable, teachers can spark students' native curiosity by making knowledge, skills, and attitudes relevant to the task at hand. They reinforce this drive, for instance, by demonstrating how new information, skills, or attitudes are applied to real problems. For example, although a student interested in radiology might not see the personal relevance in learning chart keeping on a family medicine rotation, the astute preceptor will find a way to demonstrate how this skill applies to the student's immediate responsibilities and future career. Adult learners value what is immediately applicable. Once this connection is made, the student will have no difficulty remaining attentive and motivated to learn.

Feedback

Knowledge of results increases learning efficiency in two ways: it reinforces correct responses, and it furnishes corrective feedback when the student makes an error. In addition, it may be used to motivate. I will say more later about using feedback effectively, but in general students learn best when they are allowed to make a response, are informed whether it is right or wrong, and are then told the correct answer.

Organization

New information is easier to learn when it is associated with a concept, group, principle, rule, or law. For example, if a student understands how atrial and ventricular pressure changes during the cardiac cycle, then remembering the characteristics of different murmurs is inherently easier than attempting to memorize them without an organizing rationale. Organizing information, building on previous knowledge, and linking information into meaningful categories, schemes, and principles increase what a student will learn and remember.

Repetition

Forgetting to some degree is inevitable. Memory for new information tends to decay with time, though rehearsal and practice counter this. Overlearning, particularly evident when you consider the durability of some lessons such as remembering your telephone number or riding a bicycle, proves that some things once learned are rarely forgotten. But repetition, review, and elaboration improve retention of concepts because practice shapes and reshapes the connections between facts within a network of ideas. Rote facts that have little intrinsic meaning (e.g., random zip codes, state capitals) are generally forgotten once repetition ceases.

Meaningfulness

Information has meaning when it is understandable. Techniques such as diagrams, metaphors, and demonstrations can make ideas clear. Facts that stand alone and concepts that are poorly understood are difficult to learn—it is hard to relate them to other information. Thus facts become more meaningful when they can be related to principles, ideas, laws, hypotheses, and concepts. A concept is demonstrably meaningful when students can restate the idea in their own words and use the information to solve a new problem.

Participation

Participation increases alertness and improves memory. It demonstrates an active mind rehearsing knowledge and solving problems. The best participation is overt rather than covert; that is, the student gives a perceptible response, providing an opportunity for feedback and reinforcement. Covert participation—the reflection and processing a student may do while listening only—certainly reflects learning, but the teacher cannot be sure that learning occurs if the student is not overtly participating, thus allowing assessment and direct feedback.

Support and Challenge

A supportive, challenging environment allows the learner to ask questions freely, test ideas, and propose solutions. Its value comes less from the comfort it imparts than from the opportunity it gives students to rehearse knowledge and strengthen a grasp of concepts without fear of failure or unwarranted judgment.

How can the preceptor use these principles to help students learn in a typical ambulatory medicine context?

The Teacher-Learner Interaction

It should be clear from the principles listed above that the teacher-learner interaction is a fluid and collaborative enterprise. It is not a one-way communication from the teacher to the student. At a minimum, teaching is an exchange between them (Roberts 1996). The teacher must assess the learner's needs, provide a convincing rationale for teaching the material, present facts and concepts clearly, and test the learner's grasp of the lesson in order to correct misunderstanding and reinforce the ideas. The learner must be motivated by the personal relevance of the lesson, understand what is presented, and have an opportunity to reflect, rehearse, and test the new knowledge. Thus learning is not passive—it is a collaboration that takes many forms depending on the learner's needs, the type of information to be acquired, and the exigencies of the moment. Because the settings in ambulatory medicine are so variable, the clinical skills needed so numerous, and the variation in learners' abilities so wide, the teacher must be able to adapt these principles to a range of teaching methods. (Indeed, this is part of the challenge and appeal when teaching ambulatory medicine.) These principles hold true whether you deliver a lecture, demonstrate a technique, moderate a group discussion, or supervise a student's independent study. A teacher who conceives the task as simply talking, without regard to the learner's interest, has little more chance of teaching effectively than one who simply goes about his own business while answering the student's self-guided questions. Of course the teacher may assume, based on experience, what the learner wants or needs to know and hit the mark—or not. Furthermore, there is nothing to guarantee that the inexperienced learner knows what to ask or is picking up the salient information. Only through work characterized by two-way communication can the teacher and learner effectively meet relevant and agreed-on goals.

Therefore it is a bit misleading to break apart the constituent parts of the teacher-learner interaction and analyze them separately. Doing so implies being centered on giving or receiving information, when in fact the learning process—particularly in clinical teaching—is an interactive exchange. Shifting the equilibrium too much to the teacher or the learner gives the impression that the responsibility lies with one or the other. In reality both share accountability for achieving a common enterprise—assisting the learner and making the experience satisfying for both. Particularly in the fluid ambulatory setting, where the teacher and learner remain vigilant for learning opportunities and must employ flexible teaching tactics, there is an ebb and flow as there is with any true discourse.

This said, the components of the teacher-learner interaction are communication, the learning method, the environment, and the content. This division is useful only to help analyze practical teaching situations.

Communication

The teacher's act falls within a spectrum of *telling* (e.g., sharing information, lecturing, answering questions, and demonstrating) and *asking* (e.g., probing the learner's knowledge and reasoning with open and closed questions). Telling places the teacher in an overtly active role relative to the student. The student becomes the receiver, though not necessarily a passive one. In truth, even the learner who appears to listen passively is actively attending to the speaker's words or actions. Rather than absorbing information inertly, the student is organizing it and placing it within a structure of previously attained knowledge. The teacher must encourage this procedure by preparation, providing clear meaning, organization, feedback, and reinforcement. Of course active participation enhances the effectiveness of the teacher's telling.

Asking also puts the teacher in an active role. Meaningful, nonthreatening questions engage the learner and stimulate thinking. Thus it is useful to understand the purpose of questions.

Teachers ask questions for two basic reasons: to ascertain knowledge and to stimulate thinking. Questions may take a closed or open form.

Closed questions are meant to elicit factual knowledge (Foley and Smilansky 1980). By asking closed questions the teacher may determine what a student's knows or have her rehearse information. Responses to closed questions are limited and may take the form of yes/no, listing, identifying, explaining information, or defining.

Yes/No

"Will adding digoxin to this patient's therapy for heart failure promote his longevity?"
"Does oral iron cause a false-positive stool guiaic test?"
"Is a normal oxygen saturation reliable evidence against pulmonary embolus?"

Listing

"What are the causes of microcytic anemia?"
"Tell me the causes for palpable purpura."
"List the common difference in depression between young and old patients."

Identifying

"Identify the parts of the vertebral bone shown on this drawing."
"Show me the jugular waves on this patient."
"Point to the sensory areas for the median, radial, and ulnar nerves on your hand."

Explaining

"Explain the difference between 'tachypnea' and 'dyspnea.'"
"Tell me how the pulse oximeter works."
"Explain why patients with edema might have increased nocturia."

Defining

"What is the definition of delirium?"
"Define tremor."
"What is the meaning of 'apraxia'?"

Because the answers to closed questions are limited and may rely on recall alone, they are said to tap "lower-order" thinking—the student may not be required to reason to produce an answer. To whatever extent reasoning is used to answer them, closed questions are useful for determining the learner's level of knowledge and reinforcing important basic information that is needed for "higher-order" critical thinking such as problem solving. In other words, a student needs a basic repertoire of factual knowledge to reason with. Asking closed questions can help the teacher assess recall and help the student rehearse and solidify knowledge.

Open questions require more expansive answers and are more likely to demonstrate the learner's thought process. Schwenk and Whitman (1987) list the following reasons for asking open questions:

1. To stimulate learning and thinking:
   "Based on your experience, why do you think this patient is missing appointments?"
   "Considering the risks and benefits, tell me your reason for choosing this therapy."
2. To assist the learner in organizing and clarifying concepts:
   "Considering this patient's presenting symptoms, how would you organize a differential diagnosis—temporally, anatomically, or epidemiologically—and why?"
   "What effect does this patient's increased weight have on his cardiac function?"
3. To correct misunderstandings or faulty reasoning:
   "You feel that an examination of the carotid arteries will help you determine the cause for her vertigo. Explain how carotid atherosclerosis would cause vertigo."
   "You have diagnosed belching owing to aerophagia and are recommending an antacid. How will this alleviate the patient's symptom?"
4. To assist in showing special or obscure relationships:
   "How will these vitamin B_{12} injections affect the patient's sense of well-being?"
   "How would this medication interfere with our ability to measure the patient's thyroid function?"
5. To strengthen the learner's ability to synthesize and analyze:
   "How will this (question, lab result, physical exam) support (or refute) your diagnosis?"
   "Can you think of any diagnosis that will unify these (symptoms, lab results, physical findings)?"

"What questions can you ask the patient that will help you distinguish between functional and organic abdominal pain?"

"The patient asked how you know that her rectal bleeding is hemorrhoidal. What question might she really be asking you, and how could you address it?"

6. To correct attitudes or behaviors:

"I noticed that you were looking through the patient's chart while she was telling you about her symptoms. What message do you think this conveys to her?"

"What effect does pausing after you ask questions have on the patient's response?"

"You told the patient that her headaches are 'not serious.' How will she interpret your concern for her symptoms?"

Both telling and asking have their place; circumstances determine what is appropriate. Good teachers see telling and asking as tools and find a balance that promotes active engagement with the student.

Some individuals, by dint of personality or previous training, will tend toward telling. Telling for the purpose of transmitting basic information is necessary and useful. In general, however, it has been observed that teachers tell too much and ask too little (Westberg and Jason 1993). Doing so risks more than simply "going on" and losing the student's interest; the teacher misses the opportunity to assess the student's understanding and therefore the opportunity to provide feedback. Asking, especially when well conceived and sequenced, is the surest way to know if someone is grasping the relevant information. It promotes interest and prods students to develop autonomy and critical thinking. I will say more about telling and asking techniques in chapter 6, "How to Teach."

The Learning Method

Students' learning falls along a continuum between receiving information (e.g., attending a lecture, copying notes, memorizing, or watching a video) and discovering for themselves (e.g., independent exploration, group discussion, brainstorming, researching a question, problem solving, and defining their own goals).

Corresponding to the teacher's telling, receiving typically involves a flow of information from the teacher (or book or video) to the student.

The teacher's asking corresponds to the student's discovery. It implies, on the learner's part, a greater responsibility for determining the learning content (facts, skills, and values). Receiving information in a prepared format is called *reception learning*. It is an efficient method for presenting a large amount of new information, such as core knowledge, at the beginning of a course. Sending students out to explore is called *discovery learning*. It is ideal for encouraging them to use their own skills and fund of knowledge for tackling new problems. Material learned in this way may be more easily remembered and more useful when encountering novel problems in the future (Ausbel 1968).

Students who are accustomed to the classroom may find discovery learning disconcerting—particularly if they have little practice in using independent research to tackle clinical problems. Reception learning, on the other hand, is familiar and in some ways more comfortable. This is to be expected, but it can be overcome, as will be discussed in chapter 6.

The Learning Environment

The learning environment includes both the physical location and the atmosphere in which learning takes place. The contrast is most apparent when comparing the more predictable classroom-based talk and the often spontaneous or unplanned teaching that occurs with patients in the office. Most ambulatory medicine teaching occurs along a continuum between the two. Lectures and other forms of reception learning are suitable when the objectives are defined and prepared, though telling and demonstration will often arise spontaneously from opportunities of the moment. Sometimes conferences, meetings, demonstrations, and lectures are scheduled during the course of a day in the office. The most valuable learning, however, is with patients—especially when it is supervised. Forethought that comes from reviewing goals may reduce the unexpected, but you cannot prevent it, nor should you strive to. Unplanned clinical problems are in the nature of ambulatory medical care. Learning to manage these, and consequently teaching this skill, is an appealing part of ambulatory medicine.

Finally, the environment can be open or closed to inquiry. In most instances an open atmosphere that promotes the student's participation is desirable, and the teacher should encourage questions. The teacher can create an open environment by seeking the student's opinion, allowing time for reflection, and accepting more than one answer to open questions. Sometimes, however, it is necessary for a student to simply observe while withholding questions or restraining participation. An emergency that the student is not suited to treat would be one example. Another might be a sensitive moment for the patient. In these situations the patient's needs take precedence. When this occurs the teacher may instruct the student to observe but to save questions for later.

Learning Content

The learning content varies with circumstances. Presenting a defined body of knowledge in a fixed format and with delineated objectives is *content learning*. This is familiar to students fresh from the classroom and often is the most comfortable for those accustomed to predetermined goals. *Process learning* occurs when students learn from the activity they are participating in. The environment is the content, so a student who completes a preventive care flow chart on every patient learns about preventive health maintenance (Rubenstein and Talbot 1992).

Different tasks are better suited for one method of learning or the other. For instance, a teacher might choose content learning for presenting factual information such as biostatistics, the professional's legal responsibility for impaired drivers, or the evaluation and management of a pulmonary nodule. Process learning is more suitable for teaching such ill-defined skills as "telephone medicine," chart keeping, comforting a grieving patient, or reviewing medication adherence. Skills like these involve subtle details that are not easily captured by oral or written communication. This does not mean that preparation, instruction, and guidance are not provided. It is often useful and necessary to point out what skills students should be learning. In fact, this will increase learning efficiency and reduce mistakes. It is just that some skills are best learned by doing.

These four components of the teacher-student interaction can be represented on a continuum as illustrated below (see table 3.1). In ambulatory teaching, a talk about the outpatient workup of syncope, using a review article to supplement the discussion, would lie to the left of this scheme. An evidence-based computer search to answer the question, "Do antibiotics reduce the severity or duration of acute bronchitis?" or learning billing codes by filling out billing sheets would fall to the right. Most ambulatory teaching, certainly the kind that immediately involves the student, pa-

Table 3.1. Communication/Method/Environment/Learning Content

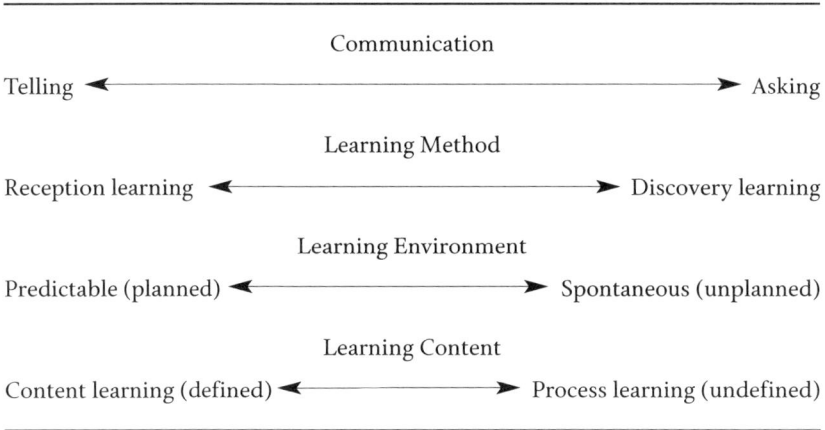

Communication

Telling ◄—————————————————————————————► Asking

Learning Method

Reception learning ◄—————————————————————► Discovery learning

Learning Environment

Predictable (planned) ◄———————————————► Spontaneous (unplanned)

Learning Content

Content learning (defined) ◄———————————► Process learning (undefined)

tient, and teacher, lies in the middle. In this case dialogue ebbs and flows, and teaching is guided by goals. Nevertheless, unplanned teaching moments occur, and the teacher can outline learning content, allow the student to learn by doing, or both, depending on the situation. The skillful teacher makes judgments based on these considerations and adjusts accordingly.

The following three scenarios represent common teaching situations one might encounter in an office. The first instance is more structured than the second or third. In the first example, even though the talk is an unplanned "minilecture," it is structured around a learner's question, and the teacher develops its content. The subsequent examples represent less structured learning experiences but are also teaching opportunities common in the ambulatory medicine environment. All three will be used to show aspects of the teacher-student interaction and the teacher's use of facilitation.

One afternoon a medical student, internal medicine resident, and general internal medicine fellow gather in the conference room of a large multispecialty practice. An internist brings in sodas and joins the group members as they relax after a full clinic day. The conversation revolves around clinical dilemmas, and the resident asks the attending physician how she decides whether systolic outflow murmurs are hemodynamically significant. When, for instance, would she order an echocardiogram to rule out aortic stenosis? She looks around—the other two also express interest in discussing this topic.

Before she begins, she asks the resident if he has a particular case in mind. He does, and he describes a patient he saw in clinic earlier that week. She then asks the three if she should start with a short refresher on the pathophysiology and distinguishing physical signs of systolic murmurs. They say yes. She uses the conference blackboard to create a cartoon of the heart and draws a chart of systolic murmurs, their auscultatory features, and response to physical maneuvers. During the talk she repeats key points, confirms each learner's understanding, and uses probing questions to confirm that they understand the hemodynamic principles she is discussing. This stimulates related questions. She rewards participation by acknowledging questions. She corrects erroneous answers and notes correct ones. To reinforce the session she offers to look at her schedule and see if any patients are coming in that might illustrate these teaching points. She also tells the group members to let her know when they see a patient with a heart murmur so she can examine the patient with them. She suggests useful reading. The resident also suggests an auscultatory skill lab at the medical school.

The group members find the talk helpful and look forward to actual supervised practice.

The entire session lasts thirty minutes.

This vignette captures many features of the teacher-learner interaction, including the principles of facilitation. This episode might be characterized as a minilecture (or a short, focused talk). It differs from the stereotypical lecture dominated by telling. Clearly there is more happening than the unidirectional flow of information from the speaker to the listener.

The physician uses telling to create a common fund of information for a diverse group. She establishes a base of information before developing more complicated ideas. It is likely that the more advanced learner knows this information, but in the spirit of learning she gets the group's consent to begin with a basic review. From her experience and her survey of the group, she knows what information to present first.

She does not confine her teaching to telling alone—she engages the learners by asking probing questions. This tests their knowledge and gives her the opportunity to correct faulty comprehension. In addition, it prompts discussion.

The students begin as receivers (one copies the diagrams), but they become discovers when they test their knowledge, search for additional resources, and find patients. For instance, when she asks them to predict the effect a certain physical maneuver will have on a murmur, they must use their new understanding to solve the problem.

Like many case-based clinical discussions, the talk was unplanned, yet the teacher quickly organized the information she wanted to present. This particular session may or may not have met preestablished learning goals, but it clearly fulfilled a reasonable need identified by the students. The goal—to solve an immediate clinical question—was therefore identified and shared by the group. The environment was relaxed and open to exploration. The preceptor encouraged and rewarded participation.

She delineated the content and presented the students with facts (content learning); however, in the future they will become adept at evaluating systolic outflow murmurs and learn by applying this knowledge to everyday clinical practice.

The teacher assisted this learning experience by:

1. Preparation. She ensured their readiness by determining previous learning and preparing the members of the group by establishing a common base of facts.

2. Motivation. She noted that the students had an intrinsic motivation to know and, perhaps, created a "need to know" by focusing the discussion on solving an actual medical question.

3. Reinforcement. She acknowledged participation, corrected errors, and provided a positive reinforcement for correct answers.

4. Organization. She organized the information in several ways, such as using a simple anatomical cartoon, a visual chart, and diagrams of the murmurs.

5. Repetition. She kept her points straightforward, avoiding the temptation to make comments unrelated to the subject (e.g., discussion of aortic stenosis symptoms). She reiterated key points in the middle of her discussion and summarized them again at the end.

6. Meaningfulness. She made the information meaningful by using

understandable concepts. She tied case-based facts to intelligible pathophysiology and the physical exam to meaningful problem solving. This increased retention of these concepts.

7. Participation. She encouraged active participation and even made the learners responsible for exploring the question on their own. She gave them suggestions for reading and using other resources and assigned them to find cases that could be confirmed and reviewed with her.

8. Supportive environment. She entered and helped establish an environment that was friendly and comfortable. However, she heightened the atmosphere of alertness by keeping the group engaged with probing questions.

This vignette illustrates just how dynamic the teacher-student interaction can be. Good teaching is rarely static. The teaching encounter frequently shifts along a continuum, using elements of telling and asking, reception and discovery learning, and varying degrees of content and process learning. The example given above also demonstrates how the successful teacher can promote learning using the teaching principles. Wherever on the spectrum the interaction is found, good teachers use the principles like tools, constantly monitoring learners' needs and reacting accordingly.

The next vignette illustrates a common teaching encounter that occurs in the presence of a patient.

A first-year family medicine intern examines a patient with osteoarthritis. The patient has a swollen, painful knee and asks the intern to inject the knee with steroid, since this has been helpful in the past. The intern says he will ask his attending to examine the patient with him and supervise the injection, since he has done this only once before.

The intern introduces the preceptor to the patient and presents a brief history of the man's symptoms. He knows from his attending's role modeling that he should stop and ask the patient to confirm his understanding of the history. The intern also catches himself using medical jargon ("DJD" instead of "arthritis") and corrects this by using language the patient understands. The preceptor examines the patient with the student. He has the student demonstrate the presence of the knee effusion and thereby confirms his skill at physical examination. He also imparts one pearl of wisdom for evaluating joint temperature. He uses the exam to review the student's knowledge of the differential diagnosis of knee effusion as well as the indications and contraindications for steroid injection. He does this in a non-threatening manner by starting with a question he knows the intern can answer. He then gently pushes the intern's reasoning a little harder to consider risks and contraindications to steroid injection that he may not have considered initially. The preceptor continues to include the patient in the discussion, and the man clearly appreciates hearing his doctors think about his "case." While the nurse prepares the patient for the procedure, the attending and the student go to the conference room and quickly enumerate the steps of the arthrocentesis on the blackboard. They return to the patient five minutes later; the intern performs a successful arthrocentesis and injects the joint.

Just after the procedure, while the medical assistant reviews postinjection in-structions with the patient and the intern writes an office note, the preceptor takes a minute before he sees his next patient to give quick feedback and instructions. He reinforces the intern's use of plain English when speaking to the patient by specifically praising this. He also reminds him to have the lab assistant prepare a sample of joint fluid so the two of them can look for crystals after the attending sees the next patient. The intern knows that if he has additional questions about the patient, there will be time at the end of the day to discuss them.

Superficially this focused "bedside" teaching scenario appears to differ from the "minilecture." However, the preceptor uses many of the same adult learning principles, albeit in a fast-paced setting, to promote collab-orative learning. In spite of the hectic schedule, the senior clinician re-sponds to the intern's learning needs and supervises the patient's care without sacrificing office flow. While doing this he uses substantially the same teaching principles as his colleague who delivered a "minilecture."

1. Preparation. The preceptor wanted the student to achieve two pri-mary goals: to understand when steroid injection is appropriate and to safely perform a knee joint aspiration and injection. He used questions to assess the intern's knowledge and supplied necessary information.

2. Motivation. The intern had an intrinsic need to know and re-quired no external motivation. Furthermore, motivation was enhanced

because the new information and skill were immediately applied to solving a clinical problem.

3. Reinforcement. The preceptor reviewed previously learned information and thereby reinforced it. He also reinforced desirable behavior with positive feedback.

4. Organization. The learning content was inherently organized around the clinical problem and treatment; therefore there was little need to place the information within an organized structure. However, some aspects of the teaching effort benefited from organization imposed by the preceptor. For instance, the teacher had the intern outline the steps of the procedure, helping him organize his thoughts before proceeding with the arthrocentesis. There is another aspect of organization that is not apparent—the deliberate choice to teach one memorable "pearl" and reinforce one skill with positive feedback. The teacher made these points salient so the student found it easier to identify and reflect on them later. Had he bombarded the intern with too much information, the points would have been lost.

5. Repetition. The preceptor had the intern rehearse knowledge, and the learning task itself built a foundation of experience to be rehearsed in the future.

6. Participation. The preceptor assessed the intern's readiness to perform the arthrocentesis and felt comfortable supervising him. The learner gained an appropriate level of autonomy—a major goal of clinical training.

7. Supportive environment. Though it was perhaps not made explicit in the scenario, the preceptor used verbal and nonverbal encouragement to show his confidence that the intern was ready to succeed at the new skill, and he also transmitted this confidence to the patient. When he questioned the intern, he did so respectfully, in a tone that signaled no-fault learning should he have to give instruction. Also, he spoke supportively during the procedure so that the intern remained calm and unflustered.

This scenario represents one of the most useful and demanding, yet satisfying, roles of the office-based preceptor. He observes, provides immediate, focused feedback, and allows the learner to develop graduated autonomy. It is demanding because the preceptor must simultaneously judge the patient's and learner's needs and respond deftly to both. Again, although the "bedside" teaching experience seemed different from the "minilecture," many of the same adult learning principles were used.

This final example of a teacher-student encounter shows the teacher using many of the same teaching principles in a less supervised educational environment.

A senior internal medicine resident spends two afternoons a week for one month in the on-site medical center of a large continuing care retirement community (CCRC). Most of the two thousand retirees in the CCRC live independently in apartments.

The medical resident's primary interest is cardiology, and the ambulatory rotation is a required part of the residency curriculum. He has no a priori interest in geriatric medicine.

After he meets the medical center director, the two discuss the resident's personal goals and his goals for the rotation. The director suggests that since many of the resident's future patients are likely to resemble retirees in this community, he might consider making a few home visits. This will give him an intimate view of their life and time to learn their perception of care access and medical costs, as well as how they manage activities of daily living or other interests that are important to them. The resident agrees that this will be an interesting and worthwhile exercise. They outline a few specific objectives. The director reviews basic information about Medicare coverage and methods of prescription financing and gives the resident a primer on functional assessments. Later the two plan to discuss what the resident learned and how this experience affected his impression of the elderly patients he sees in the hospital and clinic.

In this instance the teacher acts almost exclusively as a facilitator. He uses a brief series of lectures to establish a core of geriatric concepts (e.g., review of activities of daily living, medical coverage for outpatient services, medication use by the elderly). These enrich the resident's basic fund of knowledge and promote his independent experience. Later, when they discuss the experience, the attending will use open-ended questions to find out what the resident learned. The learning environment will not be predictable, and the content of this exercise will not be clearly defined, but the preceptor is not concerned by this lack of structure. Based on his experience, he is confident about the resident's maturity and readiness to function as a self-directed learner. Furthermore, the learning content will be determined by the experience itself when he interviews patients in their homes, yet the predetermined learning objectives will give him a way to focus his inquiry.

Not all the principles of facilitation are applicable in this vignette—some, such as reinforcement by using positive feedback, might be limited because of the lack of firsthand observation. Those that are applicable are worth emphasizing.

1. Preparation. The attending assessed the learner's goals and background before suggesting a learning task. And as noted above, he prepared the student's inquiry by providing him with basic information that created a foundation for his exploration.

2. Motivation. The resident may not have had an intrinsic desire to know more about how elderly cope in their homes or the impact this might have on their medical conditions. In this case the attending stimulated an interest (created a "need to know") by tying the project to the resident's future plans. The task thus became meaningful.

3. Organization. The preceptor laid a framework for relevant questions that the learner could explore (e.g., learning the CCRC residents' perceptions of access to medical care).

4. Participation. Clearly the process depended on the resident's active participation. In fact the actual "doing"—contacting the retirees, seeing firsthand the obstacles they face in performing their daily activities and the adaptations they make—provided most of the informational content the resident would learn. This active participation is far more likely to create a lasting impression of seniors' concerns about medical care than a talk or even a discussion with the preceptor.

5. Supportive environment. The learner was given freedom to explore and to demonstrate autonomy, but at the same time he had access to the medical director's expertise in a follow-up discussion. The resident also received encouragement to tackle the task and discover information on his own initiative.

Summary

- Learning is a collaborative process between a teacher and student.
- The teacher's job is to help students learn. This involves preparation, motivation, providing feedback and reinforcement, organizing information and ideas, repeating key facts and concepts, making learning meaningful, promoting active participation, and creating a supportive learning environment.
- The teacher-learner interaction is composed of four parts: communication, the learning method, the learning environment, and the content.
- Communication requires a balance of providing timely, meaningful information (telling) and probing and stimulating the student's thought process by careful questioning (asking).
- The learning method involves receiving information (reception learning) and exploring (discovery learning).
- The teaching environment in the ambulatory medical setting may be structured (a planned talk or demonstration) or unplanned (the teaching moment). It typically remains opened to inquiry, though not always (a medical emergency).
- The informational content may be defined and presented to the student (content learning) or may be part of the process of doing (process learning).

4

Setting the Stage for Effective Learning

Jim, a third-year medical student, is assigned to spend four half-day sessions a week for one month with Dr. Jones, a community-based internist. The course director gives him written directions to the office and asks him to call Dr. Jones one week in advance to confirm their meeting. Jim and Dr. Jones decide to meet thirty minutes before seeing patients, giving her a chance to introduce Jim to the staff, orient him to the office, and discuss his role in the patients' care.

Dr. Jones has been in a group practice for five years, and Jim is the first medical student to work with her in the office. Few of her patients know of her interest in teaching. Therefore she and Jim decide on the following plan: she will meet with each patient very briefly and ask permission for Jim to see them under her supervision. During this brief meeting Jim will wait in her office, and if the patient agrees she will introduce him. If the patient would rather see her alone, he will read in her office. This is not expected to happen often. The plan works well; most patients are glad to have the medical student participate in their care.

One year later Dr. Jones's patients are accustomed to seeing medical students with her. A small sign at the check-in desk identifies her teaching affiliation with the school of medicine. She finds that with established patients she can bring the students into the examining room with her and introduce them. Most of her patients are happy to meet the student either alone or with Dr. Jones in attendance. She continues to meet new patients alone briefly to describe her teaching role and ask if they mind having a student present.

A supportive environment benefits good teaching. Almost as much as having an interested, competent teacher, effective teaching requires a place conducive to learning. Preparation is the key. The clinician, particularly one who teaches in the office only occasionally, will benefit from careful planning, which includes examining the setting where teaching will occur. Yet the typical community practice is designed for patient care

—not for teaching. How do you create an inviting teaching environment, and what elements is it important to consider?

Whether teaching is conducted in an office, urgent care clinic, or other location, examining the environment will be time well spent on the students' behalf. Much of this is done before the clinician greets the first student. Once the necessary components are in place, periodic review will be sufficient to maintain the right atmosphere.

Elements of the teaching environment that you should examine are:

- The physical environment and teaching tools
- The patients
- The medical staff and office personnel
- The teacher-student interaction

The Physical Environment and Teaching Tools

The physical teaching space can have a profound effect on learning. Although we might prefer to think that the substance of the student-teacher interaction overrides such considerations, a welcoming place goes a long way toward assisting the teacher. Physical comfort, along with a positive learning atmosphere, contributes to students' receptivity. Space, lighting, sound, and temperature in a visually pleasing place are as important to teaching as they are to creating a successful patient care environment. Of course there may be practical limits on the teacher's ability to modify the office space, but it is important to consider how teaching will be done and if any modifications are practical.

As I noted in the introduction, schools want their students to learn in settings that replicate the environments where graduates will likely deliver medical care (Gruppen 1997), which helps them broaden their clinical experience beyond the hospital's corridors. Many of these sites will be informally associated with the academic institution, and the faculty will teach part time. In these settings most physicians who are recruited to teach will have established practices, with offices designed and organized to provide efficient, cost-effective patient care. Space is usually allocated for established providers. Likewise, the accoutrements of teaching—conference rooms, blackboards, video equipment, extra computer terminals, and a well-stocked library—may be luxuries that some practices have not invested in. Part-time teachers must take all this into consideration when looking at the space where they plan to teach.

Other requirements for the teaching mission may be relatively easy to implement. In most instances students will need clear directions to the site, perhaps advance notification of security (e.g., gated retirement communities, parking lots, parking garages), and a place to park. Students will welcome such courtesies as parking passes provided by the practice. These small amenities pave the way to a less stressful introduction.

Consider preparing a written description of the practice, including directions and a map for getting to the office (Steele 1997). This can be mailed directly to each student or distributed through the program director's office. Supplying written information before the first visit makes orientation more efficient and provides a reference source for frequently used contact names and numbers. In addition to directions, the instructions may include the information listed in table 4.1.

The program director's office should encourage students to contact preceptors before the rotation to confirm their schedules and arrival times.

It is important that staff be prepared to greet the student too, unless other arrangements are made ahead of time. Being greeted and escorted to the preceptor's office makes the student feel welcome. Likewise, the preceptor should be on time and ready for the orientation. Although this may seem like a minor point, an unprepared office or a tardy preceptor speaks volumes about what to expect during the rotation. A chief goal for this first encounter is to make learners feel that their needs are anticipated and that they belong.

Depending on the practice, the student may be designated an office to work from. This may be necessary in a practice where the preceptor supervises postgraduate trainees who follow their own panel of patients, but it is not typical for the occasional teacher, where all space is maximally used. Although it might seem ideal for students or residents to work out of their own offices, few practices have unused space. More likely the trainee will work in the attending physician's office, which will also serve as the headquarters for meeting and teaching. This arrangement works surprisingly well. Its value is that it allows the student to see the preceptor at work, since a large part of the learning experience includes watching the teacher organize and manage a wide range of activities (e.g., calling

Table 4.1. Orientation Checklist

Names, titles, and beeper numbers for key contact persons

Description of the office or clinic

    Location (address, maps)

    Phone, fax, and beeper numbers, e-mail address

    Parking instructions and passes

Description of the practice

    Demographic characteristics

    Most common medical problems encountered and procedures performed

    Description of the payment sources (e.g., fee for service, HMO)

    Types of services available (e.g., specialties, X ray, lab)

    Hospital affiliations

Office schedule

    Office hours

    Preceptor's schedule

    Call schedule

    Staff or other meetings

Expectations of student

    Student schedule

    Dress code

    Reminder to wear ID badge

    Brief description of patient care role

---

patients, phoning in prescriptions, communicating with colleagues, and working with office personnel). Because much of this is done from the physician's desk, the student will share this experience, clearly increasing the opportunities for teaching and informal communication. When the preceptor needs to use the office alone, another arrangement can be made for the student.

In most practices the preceptor works out of two or possibly three examining rooms. When the preceptor has two rooms, the student uses one when seeing patients and performs write-ups, checks labs, makes telephone calls, and so on using other available space (e.g., conference room, library, or preceptor's office).

Examining rooms rarely need modification. Generally a room outfitted for patient care will be the place where ambulatory "bedside" teaching occurs. Because the best teaching requires direct supervision, it is important that the room accommodate the clinician, patient, student, and in some cases, family members. Therefore it is important to provide adequate seating. Whether the student or the physician interviews the patient, everyone in the room should be physically comfortable so as not to interfere with communication. It is best to avoid having the teacher or student sit on the examining table or lean against the wall while the patient is seated. Ultimately, of course, this must be left to the teacher's discretion.

Tools for educating patients, such as a small blackboard, blank pads for drawing, and anatomical charts or models, assist in students' education as well. These investments can increase the examining room's use as a teaching resource.

A conference room is useful but is not essential unless you work with a large group of learners. It is clearly a benefit, however, to have a room outfitted with a blackboard and perhaps an overhead projector, which makes it easier to review charts or similar materials being used for instruction.

The following investments are useful, though not indispensable:

1. Blackboard
2. Overhead projector
3. Anatomical charts and models
4. Computer with Internet access
5. Books, CD-ROMs, and audiotapes
6. Video monitor and recorder

Blackboards are a good value as teaching aids. Preceptors who want to convey factual information or illustrate a concept can use them to enumerate points or create illuminating sketches, often improving comprehension. Of course you can accomplish the same objective with a piece of paper, but the blackboard is easier to use and therefore more practical. Even those who do not consider drawing to be a strength can develop adequate skill to illustrate points they make frequently. Simplicity is the key. Just as teachers can increase their effectiveness by saying less and listening more, they should use the blackboard economically—to make a few salient points.

An overhead projector is not essential for most small practices, nor is it necessary for teaching, but it too is a useful tool that can augment comprehension by making facts visually accessible. Its main utility in ambulatory teaching is to project written material that must be seen by a group. This may be a benefit, for instance, if you are reviewing a chart with a group of students (e.g., making a chart audit of progress notes, reviewing a note for content, illustrating a case for discussion). Teachers working with individual students do not need this device to review charts or other records.

Anatomical charts and models are underused teaching props. Drawings are good, and three-dimensional models are even better, though more expensive. Many times the physical exam is made clearer by referring to a handy model. Too often important skills such as chest auscultation suffer when recollection of the underlying anatomy is imprecise. Similarly, fuzzy concepts such as "low back pain" become clearer if you can review the relevant hidden parts.

Computers are nearly ubiquitous in physicians' offices; most use them for billing and scheduling. E-mail communication and Internet access are also widespread. Free e-mail, Internet accounts, and online library access are often benefits of part-time faculty positions. These have clear potential for improving teachers' and students' ability to research clinical questions that arise during teaching. Some find that e-mail communication with students helps them prepare ambulatory teaching exercises. For instance, a teacher might use e-mail to pose a clinical problem or an ethical dilemma that can be researched, prepared for group discussion, or discussed with an individual.

Increasingly, texts, journals, and educational programs are available on CD-ROMs and audiotapes. Interactive educational programs on CD-ROMs might aid in teaching cognitive, psychomotor, and affective skills. Software products and online services teach a wide range of basic science (e.g., anatomy, histology, physiology), clinical information (e.g., geriatric assessment, evaluation and management of hypertension), physical examination techniques (e.g., cardiac auscultation), and attitude lessons (e.g., doctor-patient relationship, ethical questions). Much of this information is free through the Internet and can be discovered with a little surfing. The quality of the content and the teaching efficacy of these products and services undoubtedly vary, but they have definite educational potential (Jaffe and Lynch 1996; Usatine and Lin 1998). Practitioners who are new to ambulatory teaching might consider expanding their stock of reference texts to include some of the books available on office-based teaching (see the Society of Teachers of Family Medicine Web site: http://www.stfm.org; see also Benzie 1999).

Video monitors and recorders are rarely used in ordinary ambulatory practice, and most ambulatory teaching scenarios do not require this technology, but they can be a benefit. For supervising postgraduate students, such as residents and fellows who perform much of their work independently or medical students who need increased supervision, a video record of patient-learner interactions can be very valuable (Beckman and Frankel 1994). Physicians who precept only occasionally are not likely to invest in this equipment; most who precept for a few months a year will observe learners directly. However, those who regularly supervise ambulatory teaching, especially those who supervise clinics where the learners manage their own panels of patients, should think about this investment. When a clinician contributes to a teaching program on this scale, schools should consider outfitting the office with video equipment and training the preceptor in its use (Weitzman, Garfunkel, and Connaughton 1996).

Online library service, Internet access to government and other health agencies, CD-ROMs, and audiotapes enrich offices that previously could not have afforded such abundant and timely resources for continuing education, research, and teaching. Although the core value of ambulatory teaching is the close personal supervision of a student by a clinical mentor in the presence of a patient, there is no denying the added value of these products and services. Furthermore, these tools are increasingly a part of contemporary office medical practice. Good modern practice requires that clinicians be adept at applying medical information to solve clinical problems, managing a continuum of patient care using information technology, and employing a variety of means, including interactive learning programs, to stay current. Actively using this technology during clinical practice, then, is very much a part of the lesson of ambulatory teaching.

I will say more about these tools in chapter 6, "How to Teach."

Patients

Most patients enjoy participating in the ambulatory medical teaching. The opportunity to tell their stories to an interested listener, to contribute to an educational mission, and to view their health care provider as a respected mentor can be gratifying. Patients seen by students in community-based practices typically see their physicians for the same time (or only slightly less) as on visits without a student present. Thus they gain in total contact with members of the health care team when the student participates. In most cases the added attention increases patient satisfaction.

Preparing patients in community-based practices for medical education will improve the chances of their accepting students and enhance their appreciation of the students' contribution. In the classical teaching model, where patients are seen at the bedside during ward rounds, they are accustomed to teaching as part of patient care. In major medical centers where most training occurs, patients consider this a necessary part of consulting the best experts. But they do not expect to encounter students or other trainees in an ambulatory practice that is not obviously affiliated with a school of medicine. Therefore teachers who volunteer to precept a few months a year will need to inform their patients that students will participate in patient care.

A helpful approach is to begin by identifying your affiliation with a particular school or health care institution. Tasteful signs displayed prominently in the office can accomplish this. For example, a small sign on the check-in counter might state something like this: "Our office proudly participates in training students from the Johns Hopkins University School of Medicine. This experience is essential to teach the skills they will use in the 'real world' of patient care."

If the school confers clinical or part-time faculty appointments on those who teach on its behalf, you might incorporate this title into your office letterhead or business cards—certainly if clinical teaching is a significant part of your activity. An academic appointment can only enhance the image of your practice, and it indirectly informs colleagues and patients that office visits are opportunities to teach students and postgraduate health care professionals.

There are also other ways to accomplish this goal. Patient newsletters might include an update on teaching. Periodically featuring students, and emphasizing their experience, can be helpful. When teaching is a new endeavor in an established practice, a letter is a courteous means of informing patients about this new affiliation.

The most straightforward method is to speak directly to patients about ambulatory teaching. Indeed, this is particularly important if teaching is not an obvious activity in the office (as it is for faculty practice), if the patient is new, or if teaching is a new venture in an established practice. Practices that are strongly affiliated with a teaching institution (e.g., Johns Hopkins Community Physicians, Johns Hopkins Bayview Physicians, P.A.) may need less explanation than those without such an obvious affiliation.

How and when you discuss teaching with a patient will vary with the practice situation. One approach is to have the staff ask for patients' consent when they schedule appointments. This saves the time spent explaining the student's role when patients arrive at the office. It is important that staff members present teaching positively; the wording can be rehearsed early on. Patients can be informed that the practice participates in medical education and that their doctor believes they would be good candidates for the medical student or resident to see. Of course patients should know that the visit will take a bit longer than usual, perhaps fifteen to thirty minutes longer, and that they will see the doctor too. Also, they should be reassured that, though their participation is highly valued, it is entirely voluntary and that the attending physician is happy to see them alone if they choose. Generally patients do not mind working with students as long as they know that the person in training is under their doctor's supervision and that they will see their own doctor too.

Where it is not possible or practical to secure the patient's consent when the visit is scheduled, the teacher or office staff should obtain permission before the teacher introduces the student. This may not be necessary if the patient has previously indicated willingness to work with students. When patients have no expectation of seeing a student or resident, it is best to first meet them briefly alone. The student waits outside, preferably in an office or conference room, while the teacher explains about hosting a student or postgraduate health care professional for a clinical rotation and describes the learner's role in clear, unambiguous terms, including the extent of the teacher's supervision and the estimated time of the visit. Patients are given the choice to participate or not, with friendly reassurance that their refusal will not compromise their relationship with the doctor. Few patients will refuse to participate. If they do, the student can wait in the teacher's office or another suitable place during the visit. Use discretion. If patients' problems seem delicate or sensitive, then even if they have previously been seen by a student you should offer private time to discuss personal matters. Sometimes a patient's acquiescence to working with a student seems cool. Your own insight and judgment will provide a clue to the best response. If you believe a patient feels put-upon, it is better to have the student see someone else.

When the patient agrees to see a student, it is up to the physician or staff to introduce them. In most practices the patient has a relationship with the doctor, whose duty it is to endorse the student's role in the patient's care. This should begin with a formal introduction, using appropriate titles of address for both the patient and the student. For those who have not yet graduated from professional school, using misleading titles such as "student doctor" or "doctor in training" is not appropriate. It is preferable to clearly identify learners as the students they are. If learners are doctors or nurses receiving advanced training (e.g., residency, fellowship, or nurse-practitioner degree), then it is proper to introduce them as such and explain the goal of their training. Patients deserve to know whom they are working with. They should not be misled, even if unintentionally, regarding learners' experience or qualifications. There is no ignominy in stating their status honestly.

"Mr. Jones, I'd like you to meet Mr. Smith, a medical student from Johns Hopkins. Mr. Smith will be spending a few weeks in our office gaining experience in office-based medical practice. I appreciate your willingness to let him see you. Tell him about your ear pain. Give him a chance to ask questions and examine you just as I would. This should take about ten minutes, and then he and I will examine you together."

"Ms. Jones, I'd like you to meet Dr. Smith. Dr. Smith is a graduate of Johns Hopkins School of Medicine and is now training in adult medicine at the Johns Hopkins Bayview Medical Center. Thank you for agreeing to let her see you with me. She will take some preliminary information regarding your health care, as I would. After that we'll talk with you, then she and I will perform your breast and pelvic examinations together."

"Mrs. Jones, let me introduce Dr. Smith. Dr. Smith has completed training in family medicine and is now a fellow in the Division of Geriatric Medicine at Johns Hopkins. He and I are working together in the office Mondays and Thursdays for the next three months. After he has had a chance to see you, the three of us will discuss your treatment together."

In some practice settings, usually as part of longitudinal primary care training, resident physicians or fellows have patient panels of their own. A community-based physician might volunteer to oversee the trainee's patient care. When this occurs, the trainee has met the patient and introduced himself as the primary care provider. The attending typically meets the patient sometime after the trainee does. The trainee then introduces the senior colleague as the one supervising training in this setting.

"Mr. Jones, I'd like you to meet Dr. Harvey, my supervisor. I want to tell him what you and I have discussed. If you'd like to add to or correct anything I tell him, please do. He may want to ask you a few questions too. After that he and I will examine your knee together."

Consider rehearsing one of the appropriate scripts with the learner before seeing the patient.

A variety of scenarios could follow equally valid, but different, scripts, but these examples illustrate two principles: the parties should be clearly and accurately identified, and their roles in the patient's care should be specified. How formal the introduction should be and how detailed an explanation of the learner's background and level of responsibility is needed will depend on the particular circumstances. For instance, some patients prefer to be addressed less formally, perhaps by their first names. If so, then it is clearly appropriate to do so. You should not, however, refer to the student or postgraduate trainee in an informal manner during an introduction to a patient. Using the first name may seem comfortable—and this may be fine in private—but it risks trivializing the learner's role and status in the patient's eyes.

Teaching procedural skills to a novice requires a deft touch; the teacher must assess the learner's readiness and the patient's willingness to participate. Gynecological exams, venipuncture, sigmoidoscopy, incision and drainage, suturing, skin biopsies, and casting are some of the more common procedures that are taught in the ambulatory setting. Patients are amazingly tolerant and understanding when a student or postgraduate needs to learn. Many patients, if approached with reasonable reassurance that the teacher will carefully supervise each step of the process, will allow the learner to perform a procedure. The teacher should see patients alone to discuss the procedure and the purpose of the training. If they agree, then they consent orally or in writing just as they normally would.

Dr. Kelly, a gynecologist, is precepting a gynecology resident in his office. His patient, Mrs. Jones, has an infected Bartholin's gland cyst. He speaks to Mrs. Jones alone and explains to her that the first-year resident he is working with has watched an infected cyst being incised but has not yet done it herself. He describes the procedure and asks Mrs. Jones if she would allow the resident to perform this operation under his supervision. She trusts Dr. Kelly's judgment and agrees.

Dr. Kelly brings the resident into the examining room and introduces her to the patient. After the consent form is completed, Dr. Kelly "walks" her step by step through the procedure.

The salient points are these:

1. The mentor fairly represents the learner's experience
2. He honestly informs the patient that the purpose of this exercise is to teach the resident in addition to treating her medical problem
3. He lets the patient decide without pressure
4. The patient trusts her doctor to sanction only what he is comfortable with

None of these vignettes capture every nuance of the teacher-patient-student interaction. They serve, however, to provide a working framework for introducing a learner to a patient and informing the patient of the learner's role in the patient's care.

Troublesome Patients

Not every patient is suited for every student. Aside from the minority of patients who do not want to see a student, some will have personalities that interfere with teaching. Unfortunately, litigious, argumentative, verbally abusive, bigoted, or sexist patients are a reality. How a physician handles these problems is a matter beyond this book. But it is rarely helpful to thrust an inexperienced learner into an encounter with such a patient unless she has dealt with this problem before or unless working with difficult patients is the purpose of the exercise. For most ambulatory teaching, where the goals of patient care are centered on acquiring more basic patient interviewing skills, burdening a student with such a patient is not helpful and is a waste of learning time.

A common source of frustration for learners is being thrust into an examination room with a patient whose problems are too numerous or complex for their level of training. For instance, a third-year medical student who is just learning to perform a focused history and physical exam should not see a child with severe developmental problems, asthma, and an acute respiratory infection during a brief office visit. At this stage of training the student should be given more straightforward problems to tackle. The teacher must always balance teaching opportunities, office flow, and the student's receptivity to a particular lesson. Students will learn little if they are overwhelmed. Sometimes the teacher will isolate a single aspect of the patient's care for the student to address. In the example above, the student might take the vital signs and watch the preceptor evaluate the patient, with an opportunity to discuss the patient's care after the visit. If this is not practical or if there are more appropriate problems to work on, it is better to avoid such patients until the learner is ready to organize care of this complexity.

Another common problem is the garrulous patient. This patient may not be well suited for a student who is just learning to interview patients and organize information. Again the teacher must use judgment, balancing learning goals, patient flow, and staff time. If a prime goal is teaching the learner—say, an advanced student or a resident—how to interview such patients, then such assignments are worthwhile; if not, then the student's time will be better spent with less challenging patients.

These warnings are meant not to shelter students from the realities of medical care but to remind you to consider the learning goals and the learner's skills before making a student-patient match.

Scheduling Patients

Teaching schedules vary depending on the type of work being done and the learners' experience. In typical primary care settings, medical students will see three or four patients each session, while the preceptor sees twice this number. Clinicians should allow students twice as much time per patient as they themselves would take for the same visit. Medical students with little clinical experience (e.g., third- or fourth-year students on core ambulatory rotations, interns new to ambulatory clinics) obviously need more time than more experienced learners (e.g., residents with ambulatory experience, fellows). Residents, for instance, may see four to six patients per session while their preceptors see eight. This can be accomplished by scheduling the learner to see a patient while the preceptor sees another one yet leaving an unscheduled visit following the two scheduled ones to allow for observation and teaching (Lesky and Hershman 1995). This is illustrated in table 4.2. For example, if patients are scheduled every fifteen minutes, then the preceptor and learner each see a patient at, say, 9:00. The attending and student schedule no patients at 9:15, and the open time is used for supervised teaching and discussion. The same number of patients are scheduled per unit of time. This model can be used for office visits of any duration. Early in the rotation when the learner is getting oriented, the preceptor allows for greater inefficiency by scheduling the learner to see fewer patients, leaving more time in his schedule for chart work, reading about the patients he has seen, and so on.

Another approach, illustrated in table 4.3, can be used when learners do not have their own patient schedule but see patients in the preceptor's schedule. The teacher simply splits the office visit with the learner. This works best with efficient learners such as fourth-year medical students and residents, but it can also be used with less experienced medical students. This working arrangement is useful when learners are in the office for a short time (a few sessions over one or two weeks) and building a patient schedule around them is not practical. It also works best when visits of intermediate length or longer (twenty, thirty, or forty-five minutes) are interspersed with shorter visits (ten or fifteen minutes), since this creates a little more "give" in the schedule flow. With this schedule, the

Table 4.2. Preceptor-Learner Schedule: "Wave Type"

Time	Preceptor	Learner
9:00	Patient	Patient
9:15	Supervision	Supervision
9:30	Patient	Write-up
9:45	Patient	Patient
10:00	Supervision	Supervision
10:15	Patient	Write-up
10:30	Patient	Patient
10:45	Supervision	Supervision
11:00	Patient	Write-up
11:15	Patient	Patient*
11:30	Supervision	Supervision
11:45	Patient	Write-up

*Optional: can be shifted to preceptor.

preceptor identifies a patient who agrees to see the student or resident. If the visit is scheduled for thirty minutes, the preceptor tells the patient that the learner will use the first ten to fifteen minutes to obtain the preliminary history, then will present the information in the patient's presence. The attending interrupts the student's history at the agreed-on time, examines the patient with the student, and discusses the treatment plan. After this the student takes additional time to provide patient education, write notes, or read while the attending sees the next patient alone. If the student finishes work while the attending is still seeing a patient, the preceptor can bring the student in to meet that patient and share whatever teaching points are of value (e.g., aspects of the history, physical exam findings). When there is a "no-show," the preceptor and learner can use the time, at their discretion, to do extra work, discuss a case, give feedback, or research a patient care question.

With either schedule there will be unexpected delays, emergencies, and the like. Patient flow rarely is perfectly orderly. The preceptor must be flexible and creative to provide patient care and oversee teaching at the same time. With practice, as for any skill, ambulatory medicine teachers find a workable balance.

Many preceptors report that teaching adds thirty to sixty minutes to an average clinic day. The extra time is spent supervising the learner's patient care, providing feedback, giving "minilectures," and the like. Experienced ambulatory teachers are not necessarily less productive, though. Most have discovered ways to increase efficiency and even find that students become assets to their productivity (e.g., writing notes, filling in medication lists, researching patient care questions, calling patients with test results). In addition to working the schedule wisely, experienced teachers use tactics that make efficient use of clinic time and turn teaching into a plus:

Table 4.3 Learner Seeing Patients in Preceptor's Schedule

9:00	Patient (new)*	Learner takes preliminary history**
9:20		Preceptor examines patient with learner
9:40	Patient	Learner completes notes/reads or joins preceptor for focused learning
10:00	Patient	Preceptor observes learner or they examine patient together
10:20	Patient	Learner completes notes/reads or joins preceptor for focused learning
10:40	Patient	Learner observes preceptor or they examine patient together
11:00	Patient	Learner takes preliminary history/preceptor supervises exam
11:20	Patient	Preceptor sees patient/learner completes notes or joins preceptor for focused learning
11:40	Patient	Learner takes preliminary history/preceptor supervises exam
12:00	Patient	Preceptor sees patient/learner completes notes or joins preceptor for focused learning

*Patient schedule: new patient, forty minutes; return, twenty minutes.

**Preceptor uses time to supervise visit or complete other work (e.g., make telephone calls, update charts).

1. Prepare the student to see the patient. Note key points in the history and suggest questions the student should ask about the history and differential diagnosis.

2. Give the student specific guidelines for focusing the exam and the amount of time to spend with the patient (e.g., "Take twenty minutes to examine this patient with rectal bleeding. Remember to check supine and upright blood pressure, examine the abdomen, and perform a rectal").

3. Have the student present the history in the patient's presence. This increases the preceptor's time with the patient and improves the accuracy of the history. Patients' satisfaction is also improved, since they spend less time alone and more direct attention is given to their problems.

4. Make patient education part of teaching the student—address discussions of the diagnosis and treatment plan to both the student and the patient.

5. Allow students to record chart notes and other data, such as updating medication sheets and primary care flow sheets.

6. Have students perform tasks such as patient education, responding to telephone messages, researching patient care questions, and tracking down results.

The Medical Staff and Other Office Personnel

Medical staff constitute a valuable teaching resource. Both professional and clerical personnel can be recruited to assist in educating health care students. Front and back office activities, depending on the goals of the rotations, are often worth incorporating into the learning experience. These may include work in the reception, billing, charting, and office management areas. Laboratory personnel, medical assistants, nurses, and other staff are often called on to contribute to the student's experience.

If you introduce teaching into an established ambulatory practice, it is helpful to meet with the staff and outline the benefits and demands that office-based teaching will entail. Teachers should not underestimate the readiness and ability of their health care teams to contribute; neither should they underestimate the burden teaching may impose on staff time, though this burden can be reduced by planning. The staff needs to understand the student's or postgraduate's capabilities and limitations, know what is expected of the learner, and know to whom they should report potential problems. Clearly, a staff member who is responsible for a significant amount of teaching will need guidance for recognizing goals and evaluating learners' achievement.

Once teaching is established, it is wise to include a regular review of the endeavor in office staff meetings. The staff should be asked for feedback; you will want to know the learner's effect on office flow and the staff's efficiency. Also, you will want to know what patients report to staff about the teaching experience—what has been positive and what has not. Do not let your enthusiasm for teaching suppress honest assessment of students or their impact on the office. It is also important to recognize that patients frequently tell staff if they are dissatisfied with care when they are reluctant to tell their doctors. This is true for all aspects of office operation and no less so for teaching. Staff, for example, may learn that a patient felt there was too little opportunity to speak to the doctor alone. Some people may tell the staff about problems with the student before they have a chance to speak to the clinician. Although this may occur infrequently, it illustrates that staff members sometimes learn important information that the preceptor should know. The teacher must have a mechanism for monitoring such feedback. Regular review during office staff meetings can improve the quality and acceptance of office-based teaching.

As I mentioned earlier, teaching can be a burden on the staff's time. Students may slow patient flow, or staff members may be directly involved in student instruction. It is important to allow them adequate time to perform their usual duties in addition to the time required for teaching. This should be fairly recognized, though monetary compensation is not always necessary, since there are many effective ways to demonstrate appreciation. But teaching should not be allowed to slow office work and require unnecessary overtime. Remember that teaching will be gratifying as long as patient flow and staff satisfaction are not compromised (see chapter 7).

Welcoming students into a practice begins with introducing them to the office staff. This is important even if they will not work directly with all members of the patient care team. Physicians do not always realize that their position can be inherently intimidating to the very people they work with and depend on. In spite of an effort to show courtesy and acknowledgment, some members of the office team may feel—whether justified or not—that their work is not fully appreciated or its demands understood. Introducing staff and treating them as valuable members of the ambulatory practice is just one way to address this need. Allowing members of the front and back office to demonstrate how their work supports patient care offers an important lesson for the student as well as giving the staff a chance to enjoy the same fulfillment that any teacher feels. The ambulatory setting, no less than other venues of health care, depends on a team to successfully accomplish its mission. In order to become competent ambulatory care providers, students must see their role models collaborating within this context.

Of course preceptors must work out teaching responsibilities with office colleagues. To the extent that teaching has an impact on their practices, the preceptor must make appropriate adjustments for productivity, staff support, and call.

The Teacher-Student Interaction

The first meeting between the teacher and student sets the tone for future interaction. Ideally the teacher transmits personal warmth and enthusiasm for the work. The approach need not be effusive, just genuine. Students rank the teacher's showing regard for them as important for successful teaching. It makes them receptive to communication and also creates the foundation for trust and acceptance when the teacher later provides feedback.

The best practice is to set aside time (usually fifteen minutes will do) to introduce yourself and learn about the student. You will need another fifteen minutes or so to show the student around the workplace and introduce the office staff. The main purpose is to welcome and orient the learner. Another thirty minutes or so can be scheduled later for discussing educational goals and developing a learning contract.

What do the teacher and student need to learn about each other? Beyond the initial greetings, the student should hear about the teacher's medical background, why the practice is enjoyable and challenging, and why the clinician wants to teach students. The teacher should feel free to discuss her own strengths, such as areas of expertise, as well as areas she has not mastered (e.g., a lot of experience suturing, little experience performing endometrial biopsies). The feeling should be that the student is being invited to embark on a worthwhile journey with an interested guide rather than standing on the sidelines to watch—and possibly getting underfoot. It is the invitation that is most important. Overcoming students' natural fear of being in the way or not knowing where they fit into the physician's practice is the point of this introduction.

A brief rundown of the schedule—giving a feel for the typical day—is an important part of orientation. Some practices have the student run through the check-in process to learn firsthand how the office works. This is also a good way to meet key personnel. Expectations about punctuality and dress should be stated up front if this is not covered in written orientation material. It is universally helpful to explain ahead of time how you intend to introduce the student to the patients. Working through the likely script, as I noted before, is beneficial. You should tell the learner that some patients might prefer to see you alone and work out how to use this free time, saving unnecessary embarrassment.

As with any learning situation, it is important not to overwhelm students with information. Most people cannot retain a cascade of new names, places, office functions, and educational tasks. Brief introductions and an overview are better. Once you welcome the student and provide an orientation to the practice space, you can set up a separate time to review educational goals.

What interests the student? What does he enjoy about patient care? Is he looking forward to learning about specific areas such as history taking, physical examinations, or special skills? What clinical experience has he had, and what procedures is he comfortable performing? In addition to educational background (undergraduate education, clinical rotations, etc.), what about long-range plans? Experience using the computer, researching medical literature, dictating, and so forth? Outside responsibilities and major extracurricular interests? Would the student or resident like to make hospital rounds, home visits, or accompany the attending as outside professional activities come up? What about learning style? Is the student a visual or an auditory learner, one who prefers facts or concepts, a watcher or a doer? All this information creates a picture of the person you will be working with.

Some information, such as that included in table 4.1, is useful to review but is more efficiently provided in a brochure. This might include examples of the scripts the teacher and learner will use when introducing one another, the most common medical problems seen, and the procedures most often performed in the clinic.

If there is not enough time to meet before getting to work, you can make brief introductions. However, do assure the student that you will schedule time for the orientation described above.

In most instances the orientation should include a period when the student "shadows" the preceptor. There is just too much to absorb early on, and medical students and postgraduates will feel more comfortable easing into their new learning environment. This may take a day or more for a true novice or only one patient visit for a resident, but observation will transmit volumes about the office procedure and the teacher's clinical style. You can use this time to introduce the student to the charts and record keeping, dictation if used, consult forms, billing sheets, working with the medical assistant, the laboratory, and other services.

Once the student feels comfortable enough to see a patient, you should start, if possible, with a problem that is likely to result in success. The teacher's intuition and experience must determine this. Novices—medical students making the transition from the classroom or early clinical years—need to develop basic communication and physical exam skills and to manage relatively simple problems. For instance, a beginning student may have a goal as basic as identifying the chief complaint and developing a differential diagnosis. If this is the goal of the visit, instruct the student to stop at that point and present her findings. Adding more to the task may be overwhelming. Clearly, some students demonstrate more aptitude than others and advance quickly, but it is usually best to start novices with straightforward patients. This allows them to adjust to the "mechanics" of the office—the most basic learning goal. From this point, once they are enjoying success, the teacher can present them with more difficult patients and more tasks per patient.

More advanced students benefit from this same graduated success. Of course medical students with experience and postgraduate students can tackle more complicated cases than beginners can, but the venue is still unfamiliar and medical skills do not always transfer easily, cognitively speaking, to new environments. For instance, residents may not recognize symptoms of cholecystitis in the office even if they would know the identical symptoms in a hospitalized patient. Furthermore, even when residents identify the problem correctly, they may be puzzled about how to proceed. Do they send the patient immediately to the hospital emergency room or first arrange for outpatient ultrasound? New environments require new learning—there is no substitute for time and experience. Therefore it is better to start slowly. You can ease the anxiety that accompanies this transition by giving all students, advanced and novice, an opportunity to build on successful encounters. This rarely takes more than a few sessions.

In short, a welcoming office whose staff is prepared to host a student will create the learning environment necessary for ambulatory medical teaching. The preceptor who plans to supervise students for one rotation a year, or at most a few, must find a workable method to simultaneously teach and see patients without significantly disrupting the practice. By planning ahead, making sensible accommodations within the schedule, and using the methods of experienced ambulatory teachers, you should find ambulatory teaching rewarding and even an asset to the practice.

Summary

- Most offices can easily integrate a student or resident into the practice schedule.
- To begin ambulatory teaching, offices need little equipment that is not already used for patient care.
- Orientation is the key to creating good rapport among the student, staff, and preceptor, and this process starts before the student arrives.
- Experienced ambulatory teachers use commonsense methods to integrate student teaching into the patient care schedule.
- Most patients enjoy participating in student teaching and report greater satisfaction with their care.
- Students do not need to see every patient; cases can be chosen to maximize the learning experience.
- The medical office staff is an important teaching resource, and staff members' input and feedback are valuable.
- The first meeting between the preceptor and student sets the tone for the rotation. The preceptor must be prepared and must use the initial sessions to gradually introduce the student into what could be an overwhelming experience.

5

What to Teach

After an office-based elective, a medical student reflects on an interviewing technique he learned from the preceptor.

A young man was experiencing recurring attacks of abdominal pain and had seen several doctors during the preceding year before consulting the student's preceptor (a gastroenterologist). The clinician took a thorough history, performed a complete physical, and reviewed the patient's medical records. The medical student and preceptor stepped outside and discussed a differential diagnosis that included psychosomatic illness, but the specialist thought the patient might have been reluctant to discuss sensitive personal information that would become part of the medical record. Before the two reentered the consultation room, the preceptor discussed a method of nonverbal communication that he uses to signal his willingness to listen to information "off the record."

He took the patient into his office and pulled his chair from behind his desk so he could sit directly in front of him. He then told the young man that before he could determine the cause of his pain, he needed to learn more about the effect of the pain on his personal life. As he said this, he closed the chart and put his pen down on his desk. The student was impressed by the result: the patient opened up and spoke freely about worries he had not discussed earlier. The communication through "body language" clearly worked.

During the first month of her senior year, a medical student is assigned to work with a geriatrician as part of a core ambulatory medicine rotation. She has an undergraduate degree in engineering and plans to apply for an orthopedic residency in the spring. She is engaged, and she and her fiancé, a medical student applying for a radiology residency, are entering the couple's match.

Toward the end of the rotation she begins to reconsider her career choice. She sees the impact a career in surgery might have on her decision to raise a family. Furthermore, she discovers a previously unrecognized interest in outpatient adult medicine. The geriatrician's satisfaction in analyzing a wide array of medical and functional problems appeals to her. She even finds personally rewarding the positive patient outcomes gained from such skills as care coordination. She discusses these ideas with her preceptor on several occasions. Later she decides to switch from surgery to internal medicine.

A pediatric resident, nearing the end of her training, requests time to learn how a well-run pediatric practice works. She wants to meet with an experienced practice manager and learn more about setting up and running a busy office. She speaks with her program director, who helps her contact a preceptor in a respected community-based practice. With her program director's help, she formulates specific goals. She will spend half a day with the receptionist handling calls and appointments, half a day with the triage nurse, and a day with the billing clerk. She will also spend two days with the office manager discussing issues such as hiring, personnel evaluations, supplies, record keeping, and compliance with laboratory regulations, among other important office functions. The information will be especially useful when she evaluates practice opportunities.

The physician who is confronted with the question "What should I teach?" might be excused for replying, "Why, medical knowledge and skills, of course." Yet experienced clinicians know that medical training requires more than imparting knowledge or even technical skill, for medicine, while dependent on these, cannot be reduced to either. It is a profession, and therefore a way of life (Bennett and Plum 1996). Thus the teacher, particularly one working in the ambulatory setting, is transmitting both knowledge and skills in the context of human-to-human interaction with patients, within a practice and within the larger society. And this, in large part, is what students need and want to know: how to put the facts and skills of medicine into practice. After years of basic science training, classroom lectures, and clinical conferences, students or young doctors want an opportunity to observe and apply what they have learned. To do this they must have teachers who are knowledgeable, competent, and capable of guiding them while at the same time delivering compassionate patient care. They must be able to teach and demonstrate problem solving. Students want advisers they can turn to, whom they can trust to listen, give consideration, and offer an informed opinion. Because the practice of medicine is a lesson in behavior, they need role models worthy of emulation, who set a standard to be followed. And if possible, they should have the opportunity to develop a relationship with a mentor who balances career with a healthy life outside the office. Not every preceptor can fill all these roles, nor is professional behavior quickly or easily learned. But it can be taught. Like apprenticeship, professionalization occurs under the tutelage of a seasoned preceptor, and the teaching is much appreciated. Clearly this is one of the benefits and purposes of ambulatory teaching—to give students a broad experience, including close contact with physicians who lead a life in medicine.

To put this in perspective you need only remember the experience of first stepping outside residency training. Even if it was very comprehensive training, you realized there were going to be many practical problems in implementing medical knowledge in an unfamiliar setting. No matter how varied and broad your experiences on the hospital's wards, the types and presentations of medical problems in the office were bound to differ (Behrman 1996). Patients would likely come to the office for conditions that would never be treated in the hospital. In many cases you would confront a diagnostic dilemma you had never before evaluated. Most problems would not be serious, but this would not always be true, and then you would have to decide, "Can this be handled in outpatient treatment, or does it require admission?" Patients treated at home would have to comply with medical therapy away from the watchful gaze of nurses and house staff. How would they be monitored and followed up?

And there would be other considerations.

Perhaps patient billing seemed far removed from clinical decisions during hospital rotations. Now income from patient care would become one yardstick for measuring your productivity. Controlling office costs, hiring and evaluating office staff, and reviewing managed care contracts might become new responsibilities.

Before, you may have devoted an extraordinary amount of time to learning. Now increased demands might be created by new family, civic, and professional duties. How should you balance these interests?

Of course, graduates fresh out of training are not expected to have mastered the skills necessary for providing excellent clinical care and running an office. They acquire them through an educational process that continues long after they leave formal training. Yet students see the challenges of a career in medicine and want to ask a senior colleague, "What did you do? How did you go about learning this? Whom should I talk to?" Teachers who have thought long and hard about these problems can share their experience with students and give advice—a necessary, valuable, and rewarding part of ambulatory teaching. Therefore teaching ambulatory medicine goes beyond the important "core" information of medicine (the cognitive, psychomotor, and affective skills needed to examine and treat patients). It includes lessons about the context of ambulatory practice (the differences from hospital-based practice), the doctor-patient relationship (patient autonomy, appropriate emotional distance, therapeutic physical contact, patient education), the mentor's personal life, and the office practice itself (its organization and management).

As I discussed in chapter 1, the goals of ambulatory teaching are many and varied. Goals will most often be defined by a program's curriculum. The learner and teacher may devise some, and still others are unstated but assumed in professional training. In this chapter I focus on those features of the ambulatory environment that are unique in the trainee's experience. I suggest themes familiar to primary care physicians, but also to specialists who practice in an ambulatory setting. These are themes to be emphasized regardless of the explicit curricular goals. Teachers should keep these in mind when working with students and use opportunities that arise during the course of teaching to stimulate and inculcate these ambulatory care principles:

1. The unique character of medical knowledge, skills, and attitudes used in the ambulatory setting
2. The doctor-patient relationship
3. The teacher's life
4. The office practice
5. The learning contract

Using Medical Knowledge and Skills in the Ambulatory Setting

Medical knowledge and patient care skills overlap with hospital-based training but differ in important ways:

1. Disease prevalence
2. Stage or severity at presentation
3. Longitudinal care

4. Treatment options and implementation

5. Emphasis on prevention

6. Emphasis on comfort, function, and independence

7. Patient-physician communication

8. Patient education, long-term medication adherence, and behavioral change

9. Reliance on history taking and physical exam skills

10. Common procedural skills

Students on ambulatory rotations soon discover that medical problems in this setting are taxing in different ways than those seen in the hospital. Hospitalized patients are typically sick and often require technically demanding care. Ambulatory patients are generally less sick, but they require many exacting skills as well. Given any time at all during an ambulatory rotation, teachers can demonstrate the expertise their practice brings to bear on patient care. Just as students learn on hospital rounds that "there are no uninteresting patients, just uninterested physicians," so they learn that many clinicians find immense gratification in performing complex intellectual tasks in a fast-paced setting. The clinician teaching ambulatory medicine benefits students greatly by imparting genuine enthusiasm for seeing the interest in virtually every patient's care, whether in making a diagnosis, devising a workable therapy, making a complex idea understandable, coordinating care, or staying abreast of medical information—to name just a few tasks.

Disease Prevalence

Typically, students fresh from the hospital have a disproportionate sense of disease prevalence—uncommon diseases seem more common than they really are in the population as a whole. This presents a question that students are just learning to face: how to incorporate the low pretest probability of unusual illnesses into diagnostic and screening strategies while maintaining a perspective on managing ordinary problems every day. Therefore an important goal is to help students learn about the illnesses most frequently seen in the ambulatory setting. They should also know the usual causes and management for common syndromes (e.g., dizziness, back pain, cough) and recognize "red flags" that warn of dangerous exceptions.

A patient comes to a physician's office with positional vertigo and normal hearing. The student develops a reasonable differential diagnosis and correctly identifies the most likely disorder (benign positional vertigo) but wants to recommend an ENT evaluation to rule out acoustic neuroma. Her attending asks her to assign relative pretest likelihood to benign positional vertigo and acoustic neuroma. She checks her estimates with a reference text and uses this information to determine the likelihood that audiograms and nystagnograms will change her clinical diagnosis. Later the two discuss how different settings (e.g., primary care clinic versus specialty clinic) influence estimates of disease prevalence.

Stage and Severity

Just as disease prevalence in the office setting differs from prevalence in the hospital, so too stage and severity at presentation often differ. Part of the satisfaction of ambulatory medicine lies in detecting problems early, when symptoms are subtler than they are likely to be on admission to the hospital. Students can learn how earlier detection and treatment prevent dangerous progression and unnecessary hospitalization. They should also learn how ambulatory care physicians rely on careful history taking and physical exam skills to detect and follow subtle changes in chronic disease.

A seventy-year-old woman experiences chronic fatigue that keeps her from doing housework. The second-year medicine resident's differential diagnosis of fatigue does not include congestive heart failure, because all the inpatients he has treated for it have had elevated jugular pressure and pulmonary edema. The attending discusses the subtler presentations of heart failure with the resident and refers him to a review article on the subject.

The same resident is surprised to learn that patients with severe congestive heart failure are not invariably condemned to cycles of hospitalization and discharge, as he has become accustomed to seeing for those admitted to inpatient services. During his ambulatory rotation he meets patients managed by a nurse-practitioner and physician team who rarely require hospitalization. He is impressed with the communication between the team and their patients as well as the patients' knowledge of their disease management. In addition to patient education and medication adherence measures, the physician demonstrates how he and the nurse use the physical exam to monitor patients' cardiac status at each visit.

Longitudinal Care

Although physicians practicing ambulatory medicine provide episodic care for self-limiting problems, much of their work is managing chronic disease and ensuring long-range preventive services. Even self-limiting problems often require follow-up. Thus most ambulatory care venues allow students to see the consequences of their medical decisions unfold over time. In this way follow-up visits provide feedback for clinical decisions, an experience often lacking on inpatient rotations, where hospital stays are becoming shorter and shorter. In the office the clinician gets to see what does or does not work. Other important principles such as watchful waiting, response to therapy, and regression to the mean are best taught when a student sees patients over more than one visit.

Longitudinal care includes providing continuity. Ambulatory medicine teachers should help students identify competencies that support this effort, such as skill in diagnosing and managing common problems; maintaining accurate, legible, and complete records; and using office-based triage and telephone-based care systems. They should demonstrate the value of using consultative services wisely to reduce fragmented care.

Longitudinal care also allows the doctor to build relationships with patients. It is important for students to see that the doctor-patient relationship develops in stages, maturing over time. Preceptors can show students how each stage affects the patient's receptivity to the doctor's communication. Over time students gain a greater appreciation of the patient as a person.

Students learn, too, that important information can be collected over subsequent visits. For instance, they learn that, unlike their experience on inpatient services, where they may have time to collect an exhaustive database, most ambulatory visits have significant time constraints and therefore require focused histories and physical exams. Students must use discretion and collect information efficiently, skills that physicians use to maintain efficient office flow.

A patient sees her family physician because she has developed moderately severe wrist tenosynovitis after taking up knitting. She wants blood tests done for Lyme arthritis. The student listens to the attending discuss the diagnosis and the pitfalls of using a blood test to make a diagnosis when the history and physical exam suggest something else. He recommends rest, splinting, a short course of anti-inflammatory medication, and follow-up. The patient is better on her return visit. The student shares the attending's gratification about the patient's improvement. Furthermore, she is impressed with the patient's new confidence in her doctor.

A patient schedules a thirty-minute new-patient visit. She wants to discuss several problems. In addition, she is not up to date with many preventive services. The attending gives the student guidance. He helps him identify the patient's most troubling problem and make arrangements for appropriate follow-up. The resident learns to set priorities and to reassure the patient that each of her concerns will be met while keeping to a workable office schedule.

Treatment Options and Implementation

Implementing outpatient treatment is complex in a way different from inpatient medical care. In the hospital departments are organized to provide prompt and efficient diagnostic and therapeutic services. Furthermore, there are social services to coordinate transition of care once the patient leaves the hospital. Office-based physicians do not usually have this coordination of ambulatory care so readily available. They often need to identify, organize, or even patch together services for patients. Nevertheless, although there are limitations on what services can be provided in the ambulatory care setting, finding alternatives to hospitalization has many benefits. These include reducing cost, preserving patients' comfort and orientation, reducing iatrogenic risks, and lessening exposure to hospital-acquired infection. Although the array of outpatient diagnostic and health care services is increasing, organizing and implementing them requires creative problem solving and judgment. This is an appealing and vital part of longitudinal ambulatory education.

An elderly woman with moderate dementia develops a stasis ulcer with cellulitis near her ankle. She lives with her husband, who is her primary caregiver, responsible for seeing that she takes her medications properly. The medical student who examines her in the office believes the patient is at risk for disorientation if she is hospitalized. But he also believes she needs intravenous antibiotics and skilled wound care. The office nurse puts him in touch with a case manager for the patient's HMO. They work out appropriate treatment to be administered in the home. The medical student stays in contact with the patient and the home health nurse by telephone. He arranges a follow-up office visit to monitor progress. The patient's wound takes a month to heal, and she is very grateful that she was able to remain at home. Her husband is grateful as well, since negotiating traffic to and from the hospital is stressful for him.

A fifty-five-year-old married man with no history of medical illness comes to an urgent care center because of intermittent cramping pain in the left-lower quadrant of the abdomen that began three days earlier. He has had a subjective fever without chills, decreased appetite, but no nausea or vomiting. The attending examines him with an emergency medicine resident. The resident thinks the patient has diverticulitis, and the attending agrees. The resident is inclined to transfer the man to the medical center for an abdominal CT scan and inpatient admission, but the attending recommends a trial of oral antibiotics, telephone contact, and a follow-up visit to the urgent care center. Later the two discuss criteria for outpatient management of presumed diverticulitis and perform an online literature search for guidelines. A week later the resident reexamines the patient, who is substantially improved. He discusses subsequent follow-up and arranges for the man to see a primary care physician.

Emphasis on Prevention

Ambulatory visits offer many opportunities to promote prevention, including risk assessment, counseling, behavior modification, age-appropriate screening, and primary and secondary preventive care (e.g., immunizations and aspirin after myocardial infarction). To provide good ambulatory care, students must understand the principles underlying these skills. In addition, the preceptor should ensure that they understand the value of documenting this effort in a readily retrievable format and developing a method for reminding patients when preventive services are due.

As a learning objective, an ambulatory pediatric preceptor asks students to include and document at least one element of prevention in each patient visit. For example, a medical student sees a teenage boy with bronchitis. The student asks the boy if he smokes cigarettes and counsels him to quit. Furthermore, he makes a notation documenting this discussion on the preventive care form in the chart. He also sees that the fifteen-year-old is due for a tetanus booster and administers it.

Emphasis on Comfort, Function, and Independence

Focusing on comfort and function puts medical problems in terms that are important to patients and sheds new light for students on the doctor's role in diagnosis and treatment. Learning how patients get to and from the office, incorporating home visits into patient care, and communicating with patients' family or friends about function give students a deeper appreciation of the impact disease can have on the patient's life. Students steeped in training that focuses on an acute disease model sometimes see medical problems that lack resolution as inherently unsatisfying to treat. Shifting the focus in chronic disease management to comfort, function, and independence teaches them that promoting comfort and improving function are satisfying goals in their own right.

A student examines an elderly man with chronic knee pain. He presents his findings to the preceptor, who asks him how this disability affects the patient's daily living. In addition to the usual questions about pain, the student learns to include questions about function, such as, "Can you describe how this problem affects your daily activities?" Using this information adds a new dimension to diagnosis and treatment. He gains an enriched understanding of the ambulatory clinician's role in identifying and solving problems that are meaningful from the patient's perspective. In addition to prescribing pain medication, he makes arrangements for physical and occupational therapy. In a telephone follow-up the patient says that with a lightweight knee brace and walker he can now do far more for himself in his apartment. He is grateful for the student's help.

Physician-Patient Communication

The office is an ideal place for teaching physician-patient communication through explicit instruction, role modeling, and direct observation with active feedback. The ambulatory physician needs a rich reserve of communication skills to accommodate the variety of patients encountered over the course of a day. Both verbal and nonverbal skills are essential. The student needs the teacher's guidance to quickly establish rapport with patients; take in relevant information efficiently; conduct patient and family conferences; negotiate with patients; overcome cultural, language, physical, and mental impairments to communication; understand patients' values and goals; broach sensitive topics; use and interpret nonverbal language (e.g., eye contact and healing touch); and teach patients effectively.

A student observes that her attending periodically stops while taking a history to summarize his understanding of the patient's story. She adopts and practices this technique. She also becomes cognizant that many patients benefit from the physical contact of the exam beyond its strict diagnostic utility. The attending identifies this as the healing touch and discusses how he uses the physical exam to convey caring in addition to gaining biomedical information. Feedback from her preceptor reminds her to converse with patients at eye level. She learns to use verbal responses and affirmative nods to acknowledge her interest in a patient's history. After reviewing a videotaped interview, she is surprised at how much time she spends looking away from the patient and writing while the patient is speaking. She readily acknowledges this as a problem and sets a goal to make more eye contact during direct communication.

Patient Education, Long-Term Medication Adherence, and Behavioral Change

As disease management and prevention shift increasingly to the ambulatory setting (e.g., congestive heart failure, HIV, diabetes, asthma), having the knowledge and skills to motivate and monitor long-term medication adherence becomes essential to successful care. Teachers should educate students about the prevalence of inadequate adherence, its contribution to poor health outcomes, and methods for correcting it. Preceptors can demonstrate methods for monitoring medication, such as asking open, nonjudgmental questions, checking prescriptions during patient visits, reviewing drug use instructions, and using clearly written instructions to ascertain and reinforce compliance. The teacher can help the student practice methods of counseling and patient education.

A resident attends weekly case-management meetings for a staff-model HMO. These are led by a nurse-practitioner who coordinates and monitors care with primary care providers for diabetics and patients with congestive heart failure. The resident also learns how the organization measures patient outcomes and cost effectiveness for this intensive program.

A student is impressed by how assiduously the office staff supports patients' medication adherence in a bustling family practice. There is a concerted effort by all staff members who have contact with the patients. The receptionist reminds patients to bring their medications to each visit. At check-in, the nurse gives positive reinforcement to those who remembered to bring their medications and reminds those who forgot about the importance of doing so on every visit. The physician always looks at each pill bottle while asking about possible problems with taking the drug and updating the patient's medication record.

Reliance on History Taking and Physical Exam Skills

Clinicians in ambulatory practice must develop, improve, and constantly reevaluate their skills at taking histories and doing physical exams. These are the primary diagnostic tools of the ambulatory practice physician, and they often are crucial in determining the pretest probability of disease. In most instances the physical exam is the most readily accessible and cost-effective tool for evaluating patients initially. Increasingly, clinicians understand the limitations and need for accuracy of history taking and physical exam techniques. This is an important part of ongoing medical education. Students learn that, rather than paying homage to tradition, good practitioners adopt new skills that are shown to work, jettison methods that are discredited by evidence, and use new technologies when they are superior and cost effective.

A medicine resident reads an article discussing the best physical exam technique for estimating the width of the abdominal aorta. The authors of the article compare expert physical examination with ultrasound and determine the accuracy of the physical exam. He asks his clinic attending to help him become more proficient in this skill. The two devise a plan to examine patients together, and the attending makes a special effort to bring the resident in to see patients who have had abdominal ultrasound performed.

A student learns that acute low back pain is an extremely common syndrome seen by ambulatory care physicians. She learns how physicians use the history and physical exam to determine which patients need an urgent workup and which ones can be treated conservatively.

A resident learns firsthand that auscultation is not sufficiently reliable for determining recovery from an acute exacerbation of asthma. He uses a peak-flow meter to measure response to therapy and trains patients to use this device to monitor therapy at home.

Common Procedural Skills

Family medicine residency training has traditionally emphasized competency at in-office procedures to a greater extent than has internal medicine or pediatric training. This is changing. It is important for ambulatory preceptors to consider common procedural competencies when assessing their own skill in light of a learner's needs and goals (Heikes and Gjerde 1985). The following, though not exhaustive, can serve as a checklist for evaluating a student's or resident's particular needs.

General

Measuring blood pressure
Venipuncture

Eye, Ear, Nose, and Throat

Fluorescein eye exam/foreign body removal
Cerumen removal
Control epistaxis
Indirect laryngoscopy
Audiometry
Tonometry

Gynecological

Pap smear/pelvic exam
Cervical biopsy
Endometrial biopsy
Breast mass aspiration
Diaphragm fitting
Intrauterine device insertion

Cardiopulmonary

Electrocardiogram and interpretation
Exercise treadmill testing
Chest X-ray interpretation
Spirometry interpretation

Suturing/Biopsy/Incising

Repair and closure of laceration
Lymph node biopsy
Excision of external thrombosed hemorrhoid
Vasectomy
Skin biopsy (shave, punch, or excision)
Incision and drainage of abscess
Excision of sebaceous cyst

Injections/Aspirations

Joint aspiration and injection
Trigger point injection
Suprapubic bladder aspiration, infant

Microscopy/Microbiology

Gram stain and interpretation
Vaginal wet mount/KOH prep
Urine/throat culture and interpretation
Peripheral blood smear and interpretation
Joint crystal preparation and interpretation
Microscopic urine exam

Miscellaneous

Proctosigmoidoscopy and polyp removal
Setting and casting simple fractures
Splinting sprains
Wound care
Removal of ingrown toenail
Basic X-ray interpretation

The Doctor-Patient Relationship

Students are interested in how their teachers relate to patients. The ambulatory setting forms a rich context for examining and discussing the history of the doctor-patient relationship as well as its characteristics.

The student will have the opportunity to see brief and long-term interactions between clinician and patients and will come to recognize that this relationship evolves through stages, from getting acquainted to testing the relationship and finally developing trust. The student should understand that both the patient and the physician bring needs and assumptions to the encounter and should appreciate that there are professional limits to the relationship and learn how to set them.

During an ambulatory rotation students will note that some relationships involve individual patients while others involve more than one person or even a network of family and friends.

Some topics that might be discussed include patient autonomy, the physician's fiduciary responsibility, confidentiality, professional caring, truthfulness, and sociocultural diversity.

Patient Autonomy

The doctor-patient relationship has evolved in recent decades. Whereas patients could once be characterized by passive acceptance of the doctor's authority, now they more often participate in care decisions. Unlike the hospital, where patients are acutely ill, in the office setting patients typically control more aspects of their lives. The atmosphere of the office visit allows the patient to exercise greater autonomy—as evinced by the decision to keep or cancel an appointment. Furthermore, the consumer movement in general has empowered patients to require information from their physicians, ask questions, and take greater responsibility for their choices. Thus the doctor's role is less often one of making decisions alone than of discussing options with the patient and working together to achieve mutually agreed on goals (Speedling and Rose 1985).

The preceptor can help students to

1. Ascertain patients' values and health care goals
2. Demonstrate respect for patients' choices
3. Inform patients as fully as possible about health care choices
4. Understand the principle of competency for making medical decisions
5. Understand and counsel patients about advanced directives
6. Recognize that some patients prefer to have the physician guide their decisions

Fiduciary Responsibility

Professionals have a fundamental responsibility to place the interests of their patients above their own. This is an old problem, but it takes on new twists as physicians become increasingly involved in the business of medicine. Practitioners of ambulatory medicine have not been spared these tensions and must deal with them daily. The fiduciary responsibility to patients may conflict with the physician's other responsibilities or enterprises that have a direct effect on office practice. For instance, the preceptor might discuss

1. The effect that office-based services such as laboratory, X-ray, and prescription sales have on the implicit trust between patient and provider

2. Managed care contracts that link incentives and bonuses to use of services

3. Activities, such as advertising, that promote physicians' practices

4. Drug company detailing to physicians

Confidentiality

Although the communication between the patient and doctor is generally privileged, circumstances arising in ambulatory practice demand professional judgment and, on occasion, legal consultation. The presumption of confidentiality within the doctor-patient relationship is becoming more complex. During an ambulatory rotation, students are likely to encounter instances such as these that affect confidentiality.

1. Communication about patients with their family or friends

2. Patients' rights to read and obtain copies of their records

3. Confidentiality of electronic and other patient databases

4. Physicians' obligations when patients present a danger to the public

Professional Caring

Understanding professional responsibilities and boundaries is a prerequisite to caring. The professional expresses caring appropriately—without resorting to a casualness that might undermine the patient's dignity or trust.

The professional also looks past superficial qualities or behaviors to patients' humanity. This demands patience and empathy and is especially challenging when a patient is needy, is angry, or has a difficult personality.

The preceptor can use opportunities that arise in practice to teach the student how to

1. Respond appropriately to angry, emotionally needy, or demanding patients

2. Interact constructively with chronically difficult patients

3. Meet patients' extenuating needs

4. Identify personal biases and negative feelings engendered by patients

5. Discuss patients as people rather than as cases or entities

Truthfulness

Maintaining patients' trust requires truthfulness. Keeping patients informed about diagnosis and prognosis while preserving hope is a delicate art. Students should observe and, depending on their skill level, be given opportunities to

1. Participate in explanations of diagnosis and prognosis that are difficult for patients to hear

2. Discuss the consequences of withholding medical information from patients at the request of well-meaning family or friends

3. Respond appropriately to patients who make requests that are contrary to the physician's values

The Teacher as Role Model and Adviser

Teachers must keep in mind that their students value them as much for who they are as for what they know. Personal qualities such as curiosity, caring, honesty, humility, generosity, and perseverance are of intense interest to students. Watching physicians relate to their patients and to their families, colleagues, employees, and the students themselves teaches lessons that students will absorb. Thus a good teacher is a role model in whom they see traits worth emulating. Acquiring these behavioral and attitudinal traits is an important part of professional education. Many of these attributes, like generosity, can be taught and reinforced. Unfortunately, the opposite is also true: bad traits can be taught. Unprofessional behavior toward patients and staff may teach students the wrong lessons and impart behavior and attitudes that discredit the profession.

Psychosocial Aspects of Medicine

Valued teachers stress the doctor-patient relationship and emphasize the psychosocial dimensions of medicine (Wright et al. 1998). Students who want to become competent doctors understand that biomedical knowledge divorced from a human context is often ineffective as well as unrewarding. Teachers should use every opportunity to demonstrate how to obtain and incorporate information about patients' functioning, culture, beliefs, and values that may affect diagnostic and therapeutic choices.

A second-year family medicine resident evaluates an elderly diabetic woman who has recently moved from Puerto Rico and is living with her daughter. The resident takes an extensive social history, yet her preventive and therapeutic plans do not reflect the patient's values. The attending suggests that as an exercise the resident create a list of priorities as seen through the patient's eyes. They compare the patient's priorities (inferred from her history) with those the resident had generated and see where the discrepancies lie. When the resident incorporates the patient's values into the biomedical information, she produces a significantly different set of recommendations. The exercise also helps the resident focus her patient education efforts on areas the woman is receptive to hearing.

Continued Learning

Ambulatory medicine teachers confront a wide array of problems that may generate a large number of clinical questions. Good clinicians are inquisitive as well as knowledgeable. They want to know the reasons behind what is apparent, and this too is worth modeling. Thus they take time to hear patients, readily admit what they do not know, and research unresolved questions. Teachers should have a system for applying evidence-based knowledge in their practice and should demonstrate this to students.

An attending sees an elderly woman who is suffering from a chronic cough secondary to an ACE inhibitor. The medical resident accompanying him during clinic asks if angiotension blockers cause coughing as well. The attending tells the resident in the patient's presence that he does not know but will look it up. A few minutes later the two have their answer.

A physician and student examine a healing traumatic wound on a young boy. The mother asks a question about dressings that the attending is not sure how to answer. He tells the mother he will bring in a colleague who has more experience with this. Later he and the student discuss values such as honesty in the doctor-patient relationship.

Teamwork

High-quality ambulatory medicine increasingly depends on teamwork and delegation of responsibility. Physicians, nurses, nurse-practitioners, physician's assistants, medical assistants, and other office personnel commonly work in interdependent teams. Effective, respectful communication is essential. Students exposed to ambulatory medicine will learn the value of the team members' roles through the respect shown by the mentor as well as by working directly with the different members.

Finally, the teacher's life itself is inherently interesting to students. The teacher may have negotiated decisions that the student now faces. When possible, preceptors should create opportunities to chat about their own career paths and discuss the experiences that influenced their decisions. Students frequently want to know what effect those decisions have had on the teacher's life outside medicine. Time to confer with a mentor is a precious commodity for learners, who frequently are pushed forward quickly in their career decisions. A teacher who generously gives time to discussing such issues is greatly appreciated.

Frequently asked questions are:

- How does a practitioner keep current with medical information?
- What are the merits of solo, staff-model HMO, group, and multispecialty practice?
- What are the merits of careers in the private, government, industry, and academic sectors?
- How does one balance family life and work?
- Can a generalist achieve a satisfying level of expertise, or must one specialize?
- How difficult is it to change careers during one's professional life?
- What medical societies does the preceptor belong to, and what are the benefits and responsibilities of membership?
- How does one handle requests for medical advice from family and friends?

- What does the preceptor do to remain enthusiastic about practice? How can one avoid "physician burnout"?
- How does the preceptor discuss medical mistakes with patients?
- How does one maintain appropriate professional distance in the doctor-patient relationship?

Students have many questions, and these are only a sample of those they might ask. The range and depth will depend on the quality of the relationship that develops between teacher and student. When they develop good rapport and the teacher is available, interested students will welcome the chance to explore this extra dimension of professional life. Of course, as with any professional relationship, the teacher must set boundaries and use judgment and discretion about what it is appropriate to discuss. For instance, an honest appraisal of your own challenges, disappointments, or limitations can provide refreshing insight for a student who might be puzzled by self-doubt. You should not, however, burden a student with personal problems or work-related frustration. The student is not a personal friend or counselor. Still, sharing time and experience is often one of the most memorable aspects of teaching ambulatory medicine.

The Practice

One purpose of teaching ambulatory medicine is to expose students and house staff to a model of efficient, high-quality practice that

- Promotes excellent medical care within financial constraints (cost-effective care)
- Supports employee morale and productivity
- Promotes efficient patient flow
- Promotes patient satisfaction
- Ensures the efficient flow of information between providers and locations of care outside the practice
- Maintains medical records that make it easy to retrieve information and promote comprehensive longitudinal and preventive care
- Maintains useful patient education materials
- Maintains systems for monitoring practice quality and productivity

Learning about the office operation is a goal for most ambulatory rotations. Students and house staff who have a longitudinal learning experience will learn much about office operation by seeing and doing. In some cases students will identify specific skills they would like to learn (e.g., telephone medicine, understanding the roles of support staff, record keeping, scheduling). In many instances the staff best teaches the functions of a well-run office. Also, one should not assume that office operations are obvious to the student. In addition to introducing support staff, set aside time for students to interact with those who make the office work.

High-Quality, Cost-Effective Care

Office operations and medical decisions are regularly affected by economic constraints. Students can gain an appreciation of the office budget and its effect on staff, supplies, and services by working with the practice manager. Teachers can demonstrate and discuss how costs affect medical decisions and patients' access to care. Students should be taught to make cost-effective decisions when devising diagnostic and therapeutic plans.

Employee Morale and Productivity

Students should appreciate the close interdependence of medical and clerical staff. Good employee morale and sustained productivity are necessary components of a successful office. They should see the preceptor communicate with staff and delegate responsibility. Demonstrating respect for staff viewpoints that concern office operation and patient care reinforces this.

Efficient Patient Flow

Appointment access, care triage, waiting room design, patient intake, and timely visits and check-out all contribute to patient flow. Students should have the opportunity to observe and discuss how these promote patient care and satisfaction with service. For instance, what are the consequences of overbooking? What are the advantages and disadvantages of open-access scheduling? What level of training does the staff need to triage phone messages, and how are these handled by staff? How does waiting area design affect patients' comfort? What influences patients' perception of waiting? If the practice cares for sick children, is there a separate waiting area? How long is it between check-in and seeing the provider? How does flow affect care quality and practice income?

Patient Satisfaction

Increasingly, practices are judged by patients' satisfaction with service, whether in fee-for-service or managed care models. To remain successful, physicians and staff must be sensitive to patient satisfaction and monitor it. Using valid tools for assessing and responding to patients' concerns is a useful skill that students can learn during an ambulatory rotation.

Efficient Flow of Information to Other Care Providers

Office practice requires care across a continuum of locations and services. It often takes great effort to ensure that different providers are kept informed of patient care decisions. The teacher can impart valuable lessons to the student about staying informed and informing others about patients. The student should understand the importance of

1. Educating patients to keep their primary care provider informed about changes in their health or health care
2. Communicating succinct, useful patient care summaries and preoperative evaluations to consultants and other providers
3. Making appropriate use of dictation, fax, pager, and e-mail
4. Ensuring that patient records are well copied and organized when care is transferred

Medical Records

Chart organization, including maintaining flow charts, intraoffice information, and record keeping, occupy a tremendous effort within ambulatory practices. Students should appreciate that this is done to promote patients' safety, fulfill regulatory and legal requirements, and achieve efficient information flow to providers. In primary care practices they should see how it promotes longitudinal and preventive care. Tracking systems for laboratory and test results and pending consultations are essential ambulatory practice skills. Students should learn practitioners' preferred methods for documenting that records and test results have been reviewed before they are filed, informing patients of results, and handling telephone messages.

Patient Education Materials

Patient-centered care relies on patient education to promote participation in health care decisions. Ambulatory practice increasingly uses patient education materials and techniques that extend learning beyond the time limitations of a typical office visit. Practitioners can demonstrate the effective use of these educational methods. In addition to printed material, they may include interactive computer programs, educational Web sites, and take-home reading materials and videos.

Monitoring Practice Quality and Productivity

Students can be shown that in addition to providing high-quality care, good practices must increasingly document this care. Many health systems and third-party payers require this. Peer reviews of charts for quality indicators, such as records of immunization, chart legibility, or adequate documentation of services are worth demonstrating to students.

The Learning Contract

Finally, "what to teach" is determined by the student's needs. This will differ widely for students and postgraduates—from the basic to the advanced. As I noted in chapter 1, some of these goals will be explicit and determined by the curriculum, some will be worked out with the learner, and others are assumed. However, it is always worthwhile to establish a learning contract at the beginning of a rotation.

A learning contract, just as one would imagine, is an agreement between the teacher and the student (Lowry 1997). It may be explicit or implicit, though explicit contracts are preferable. For longer teaching encounters, such as core ambulatory rotations, a written contract is best. An oral contract is usually sufficient for short teaching sessions. Whether written or oral, it should be open and negotiated with the student. In it the student and teacher determine at the beginning of the rotation what will be taught and how. Ideally, it specifies when feedback will be given. In addition to curricular goals, the learning contract should leave room for goals and objectives identified by the student and the teacher. Once a written contract has been reviewed and agreed on, student and teacher should each keep a copy for future reference.

The contract should be made part of the systematic review during the student's rotation. It should be mutually agreeable to renegotiate and modify the contract as student and teacher see fit. This will help them stay on target and result in a satisfying experience for both.

A learning contract framework that might be used during a core ambulatory rotation could include the following:

1. The student's most important goals (three is typical)

2. Specific strategies that the student plans to use to accomplish these goals

3. Activities the student would like to plan during the rotation

4. How the student would like to review these goals and receive feedback

Of course it is understood that the student's goals, methods for accomplishing them, desired activities, and preferences for feedback must be built around the preceptor's experience with what works. Clearly these must be achievable and agreed on.

Summary

- Although medical knowledge, skills, and values in ambulatory practice overlap with those of inpatient medicine, there are important differences. These differences include disease prevalence, stage and severity of disease, longitudinal care, treatment options and implementation, disease prevention, preserving function, doctor-patient communication, patient education and long-term adherence, reliance on history taking and physical exam skills, and common procedural skills. The preceptor can demonstrate how using this knowledge creates an expertise that makes ambulatory practice satisfying.

- Ambulatory care teachers should use their increased opportunities for observation and discussion to cover important aspects of the doctor-patient relationship, including topics such as patients' autonomy, fiduciary responsibility, confidentiality, professional caring, and truthfulness.

- Students appreciate teachers for who they are and what they do. As role models teachers should emphasize the psychosocial aspects of medical care, continued learning, and teamwork with staff and colleagues.

• Ambulatory practice offers a hands-on chance to learn office management skills. These include providing high-quality, cost-effective care, promoting high employee morale and productivity, maintaining efficient patient flow, assessing patient satisfaction, ensuring flow of information across the care continuum, maintaining medical records, and using patient education materials effectively.

• A learning contract should be developed that specifies what will be taught. It should include a few agreed-on, achievable goals and outline who will do what and when. It should set up a mechanism for feedback on progress.

6

How to Teach

Dr. Smith is a pediatrician in a small group practice. She sees general pediatric patients but devotes one session each week to adolescent medicine. In addition to her private practice she is on the clinical faculty of a medical school and volunteers to precept medical students, pediatric residents, and fellows in her office for core ambulatory pediatrics. She supervises about three medical students a year for one-month rotations. The pediatric residency director occasionally asks her to host a resident who would like to work in her adolescent clinic for two or three sessions. Once a pediatric fellow who was obtaining her M.P.H. arranged to spend one afternoon a week with her for a year. All three experiences have brought unique challenges and rewards. Over several years, Dr. Smith has developed diverse skills to meet the needs of various learners.

Dr. Jones finds ambulatory teaching hard work, but pleasant. In many respects it is challenging in the same way as patient care. His responsibilities include assessing the learner's needs before each learning situation, searching his "teaching tool bag," and using the right instrument deftly. Sometimes this requires listening and unobtrusive observation followed by feedback. At times the student wants a short, interactive "minilecture." Other times he finds it is better to let the student work independently, thereby gaining autonomy. Every learner is different, and every learning opportunity is different. Balancing teaching with patient care adds spice to his day. Still, he welcomes respites from teaching too, which give him time to reflect on the feedback he receives from students, prepare topics for future teaching, and consider how to implement new methods based on his recent experience. He is happy that in the short time since volunteering to teach ambulatory medicine in his office his teaching skills have steadily improved.

Dr. Rodriguez likes people. One could fairly describe him as a "people person." Therefore it is no surprise that he enjoys welcoming new students into his internal medicine practice. In addition to finding immense pleasure in his work, he likes sharing his experience with others. In fact, he is a natural salesman for his profession. Students who work with him leave with a definite appreciation of what he enjoys about internal medicine. More important, they consistently report to their course director that he takes a personal interest in them and makes sure he is giving them the experience they need to meet their goals. He has signed up for several seminars at local and national meetings to enhance his teaching technique. He also finds that the work he puts into teaching students improves his communication with patients.

"How to teach" begs the question, "What do good clinical teachers do?" Perhaps the answer can be found by studying the habits of model teachers—those whose students cite lessons and demonstrate skills they learned long after the experience has passed. These preceptors, whose teaching imparts durable knowledge, competent performance, and professional behaviors, set the standard for good teaching. So what skills do they deploy so effectively? What recognizable teaching principles do they use, and how can one apply them to the most common learning situations in ambulatory medicine?

Good teachers, whether they teach biochemistry in a classroom or clinical medicine in the office, rely on certain basic principles (Irby 1978; Ericksen 1985; Roberts 1996) that transcend the topics they teach and the settings where they teach them. They empower students to carry learning beyond their immediate experience and apply it to novel problems. Good teachers impart important information and help their students become critical, independent thinkers. To accomplish this they use skills that follow directly from adult learning principles. Good teachers

1. Know their students' needs
2. Identify and organize material (learning content) that is worthwhile
3. Help students encode and integrate information, thereby making it memorable
4. Stimulate curiosity and critical thinking
5. Enable students to practice skills and achieve appropriate independence

6. Create a collaborative partnership that allows them to correct students' mistakes and confirm their competence

Applying Principles to Ambulatory Teaching

The physician's office, as I noted in the introduction, is a highly variable teaching resource. In addition to the differences between primary and specialty care practices, students vary tremendously in experience and skill. Also, the duration of teaching encounters ranges significantly, from a few sessions with a preceptor to longitudinal experiences over a month or more. Therefore any discussion of teaching principles that are to be used in the office will necessarily emphasize general skills, while illustrations will incorporate specific examples.

Identifying Needs and Organizing Learning

The ambulatory setting is a hard place to teach—perhaps more than any other venue. It is frequently fast paced and unpredictable, sometimes chaotic, and difficult to organize for teaching. Who can be sure that a student will see a particular type of problem or encounter the right case mix? How will the teacher correct this if it is a problem? Even when teachers and students have specific goals, they must rely to some extent on the problems that patients present during a given session. On the other hand, there are so many potential lessons to be learned from every patient encounter that the teacher and student may be tempted to forsake primary goals and pursue interesting diversions. Yet students learn best when they focus their energy on a few well-defined goals. Therefore good teachers recognize their students' needs and help them to organize the information required to achieve their goals—to strip away confusing and distracting information and concentrate on a specific task. To accomplish this, they adopt practices that lessen office chaos and improve students' ability to stay on track. Preceptors should take time for these procedures:

- Review the student's goals before each session or at least regularly for longer rotations. A checklist based on the learning contract helps to accomplish this.
- If possible, select with the student a particular goal for each session and concentrate on it. This may simply be an oral acknowledgment of a

previous agreement or may be based on the student's self-assessment. ("What do you say we concentrate on ——— today?" or "What would you like me to work on with you today?")

• Avoid being distracted by interesting but irrelevant goals. It requires discipline to hold back from commenting on every intriguing feature of a patient encounter. Remember that students have a lifetime to learn; learning a few points well beats forgetting a welter of facts. Also, they need time to process new information.

• Review the schedule and the patients' charts before each session. Look for opportunities to match the patients to the student's needs (e.g., level of complexity, specific teaching points, case mix).

• Have a backup plan for downtime (e.g., patient "no-shows," patients who would rather see the attending alone, gaps in the schedule). Use the time for independent study, working with staff or colleagues, completing records, returning calls, researching clinical questions, and so on.

• Develop a pool of patient volunteers with interesting medical histories or physical exams. For instance, some retired patients enjoy spending time with medical students or residents and do not mind coming to the office or having a home visit for teaching purposes. These patients can be called on to fill teaching needs that may not be found in the regular practice mix (e.g., student sees several patients with osteoarthritis but none with rheumatoid arthritis for contrast).

• Assemble materials and teaching aids before sessions: equipment, models, charts, or cases to review.

• Make arrangements with staff to teach important skills (e.g., venipuncture, urinalysis, charting). This gives the staff time to prepare and optimize the student's experience.

• Brush up on topics of interest ahead of time. Clarify concepts, definitions, and organizational schemes before clinic. Review didactic information and practice skills needed to achieve teaching goals before the session.

• Develop a repertoire of minilectures and demonstrations for recurring topics and themes.

• Develop a file of reference articles, book chapters, Web sites, and such that can be used to teach important concepts and lessons.

Making Lessons Memorable: Helping Students Encode and Integrate Information

Memorable facts are linked to real experience and concepts. Nowhere is this truer than in clinical medicine. Facts are in ample supply; teachers who make them memorable are harder to find. Successful teachers—those who make a lasting imprint on their students—find a way to tie new information to real patients, real problems, or important ideas. They demonstrate how physicians use clinical information to solve the problems they encounter in the office. Information that lacks a connection to useful concepts or real clinical problems is usually acquired by rote memory— unfortunately, it decays quickly after rehearsal is discontinued. Facts that are related to concepts and clinical experience are more durable. Thus good teachers help students encode new information and integrate it with organizational schemes, principles, laws, and experiences. For instance, if the statement "Diabetics suffer a high rate of reactivation tuberculosis" is made in isolation from a specific clinical experience or is given no conceptual rationale, then it will likely be forgotten unless it is recalled frequently. The statement "Diabetics are immune suppressed with respect to tuberculosis and therefore suffer a higher rate of reactivation tuberculosis than nondiabetics" is more memorable because it links a fact to a concept. By learning the rationale—making sense of the information—the student relates the fact (diabetics suffer a higher rate of reactivation tuberculosis than nondiabetics) to an explanatory concept (immunosuppression). This works because new information that is organized within mental networks is more easily related to similar information (e.g., diabetics with positive tuberculin skin tests should receive antibiotic prophylaxis). Once this information is related to previously held knowledge, it is rehearsed and reinforced as new information is attached to the network. It is also easier to retrieve.

Furthermore, patient care provides instances for rehearsing mental models. New experiences are related to past experiences. Thus the student places new experiences within a conceptual network (e.g., diabetic–positive tuberculin skin test–immunosuppression). By building a network of concepts, experience, and information, the student recalls solutions to past problems and becomes a more efficient problem solver.

More than serving as repositories of facts, students want teachers who transmit principles and concepts and put them into practice. This is the most valuable expertise that ambulatory teachers can provide.

• Whenever possible, teach based on real experience with patients. If necessary, use case-based lessons from recent encounters, real problems based on chart review, or other concrete examples. Avoid relying on a lecture format; look for ways to use patient care to teach the same points. For example, if a student wants to learn about pain management in osteoarthritis, a preceptor could choose to answer the question by delivering a short talk. But finding a patient with osteoarthritis and using this exposure to teach about pain management will be more effective. If such a case is not immediately available, the teacher can suggest delaying the discussion until they see an appropriate patient. This is certainly feasible for common problems. An alternative is to have students describe a case from their own experience and build a short talk on that example. Likewise, teach from concrete examples that present during clinic; avoid stating facts that are not immediately relevant to the clinical problems at hand. For example, it is far more meaningful to say, "There are three reasons for liver enzymes this high: viral infection, drug toxicity, and anoxic liver damage" while examining a jaundiced patient with elevated liver enzymes than to pull this fact out of thin air while examining a healthy patient's abdomen.

• Define terms as unambiguously as possible, and state concepts clearly. Terms and ideas that cannot be articulated well are hard to remember—they cannot be placed in a mental scheme. Furthermore, they are harder to apply to novel cases. Learn to state definitions of common or important diseases, symptoms, syndromes, and the like as accurately as possible. "Vertigo is the illusion that a person is moving relative to his environment" is preferable to the more imprecise statement, "Vertigo is a type of spinning dizziness." The student who grasps the first definition will have less difficulty generalizing from it and recognizing vertigo in its variant manifestations. Furthermore, allow students to rehearse definitions orally. Having them define terms and concepts before discussions helps them acquire new information.

• Teach concepts and principles when possible. Adults prefer to learn themes and ideas that tie information together rather than to accumulate plain facts. Furthermore, basic unifying ideas are remembered longer. For instance, when examining a bunion, after defining the abnormality it is good to say, "Bunions result from excessive laxity of the metatarsal joint, most often associated with hyperpronation of the ankle." By learning this principle, the student will immediately recognize why an orthotic device that corrects hyperpronation is used in the long-term management of the problem.

• Students prefer different styles for learning concepts—visual, auditory, experiential, or abstract. Use drawings, metaphor, role playing, or other techniques to bring lessons and experiences alive. Discussion is fine, but it may not be enough.

• When teaching, limit new information or teaching points to five or fewer. Retention of new information is poor to start with, and most people cannot manipulate more than this in short-term memory. Enumerating discrete facts will also help students keep track.

Consider these teaching principles using the following examples:

A third-year medical student sees an eighty-year-old woman who has fallen several times in the past few weeks. The patient's chief complaint is chronic back pain that interferes with her sleep. Two family members give conflicting reports about her alertness. There seem to be several problems: back pain, falls, and delirium. The medical student knows the differential diagnosis for each of these, but she is having difficulty piecing together a coherent history. Consequently she cannot construct an explanatory hypothesis that accounts for the woman's symptoms. The attending helps the student conceptualize the problem as a chain of causal events. He shows her how to construct a time line that displays the woman's symptoms and links seemingly disparate parts of the history—the long-standing, unrelieved back pain, taking more over-the-counter pain medications and sleeping remedies and adding new ones, sleep deprivation, and ultimately delirium and falls. As important as the case might be for discussing the differential diagnosis of back pain, falls, or delirium, the student values the new concept of developing a time line for viewing the patient's history. Furthermore, she creates links between the elements of the history—pain, medication, sleep deprivation, falls, and delirium—that she will reinforce whenever she encounters one of these problems and recalls this experience.

A family practitioner and a third-year resident examine an otherwise healthy thirty-year-old woman who has mild anemia and low MCV. The resident suggests an anemia profile, including a serum ferritin level. It is clear that he knows a lot about anemia. It is also clear that during his hospital rotations he has learned to get a complete workup on all anemic patients. He seems to consider only how the lab tests will support his diagnosis rather than what effect they will have on his clinical decision. In this case the attending could discuss the prevalent causes for iron deficiency in various patient care settings. However, he can also use this opportunity to teach a more broadly applicable principle. He can demonstrate what he thinks about the possible outcomes of ordering tests and how he will use the tests to discriminate among alternative hypotheses. The student learns to ask himself before ordering lab work or other tests, "What effect will this test have on the patient's care?"

A student on an ambulatory pediatrics rotation tells the supervising physician about a fussy child with a minor URI. The pediatrician recognizes that the mother brings her child to the doctor a lot. In addition to discussing medical treatment of URI symptoms in infants, she points out that unusually frequent visits should trigger certain medical and psychosocial questions (looking for patterns). The student thinks about this principle on future rotations as well.

Stimulating Curiosity and Critical Thinking

Acquired facts are one measure of learning. But as important as a good fund of knowledge is, learning to use the information is the crucial skill of good physicians. Thus, stimulating students' interest in solving problems and giving them the skills to do so is a prime goal of ambulatory teaching. Clinical problem solving requires gathering and organizing information, building hypotheses, evaluating alternatives, implementing a working plan, and testing—all higher-order processes. One way to encourage this approach is by asking questions. Probing, open-ended questions that are logically sequenced help develop thinking skills (see chapter 2). Asking well-phrased questions requires practice and perhaps coaching from colleagues.

- Students are often shy about committing themselves and putting ideas forward. Prepare students to receive and answer questions. Make them aware that questions, particularly open questions, will be an integral part of learning. Reassure them that they will not be embarrassed and that "right" answers are not as important as the thinking behind their responses. During orientation, review the types of questions (see chapter 2) and explain how they will be used.

• Studies have demonstrated that the vast majority of the teacher-student interchange is factual and that most questions are lower-order ("yes/no," rote facts) rather than higher-order ("Why do you think...?" "How do you tie together...?" "Explain why you chose..."). Resist the temptation to supply answers. Choose a mix of open and closed questions to adequately assess the learner's knowledge and thinking.

• Avoid questions that telegraph answers—so-called leading questions—which preclude students' articulating independent thought. Avoid questions such as, "We're dealing with sciatica, aren't we?" "I don't think his chest pain is angina; what do you think?" In both cases students are hard pressed to disagree and can offer only one possible answer—yes or no. Moreover, they are not being asked to defend an opinion and provide supporting evidence.

• Set aside time for probing questions that follow a Socratic format. The teacher asks an open question such as, "You suspect that the patient has irritable bowel syndrome. What about her history led you to make this diagnosis?" The learner's answer then leads the teacher to explore the reasoning in more depth. ("Yes, I see your point. What aspects of her history are unusual for irritable bowel?" And so on.) Asking a sequence of probing questions can be time consuming and therefore difficult to do during a fast-paced office flow. Still, this is a valuable exercise. Good times to explore a few problems in depth usually occur during breaks or at the end of the clinic day. Discussion often ensues.

• When asking questions, give students adequate time to answer. Pause. Then pause some more. It is not uncommon for teachers (or physicians interviewing patients) to impatiently follow a question with an answer. Let students think, then answer, even if the answer is wrong. They will soon learn that they are not passive receptacles for the preceptor's fount of information.

• Clinical questions commonly arise in the course of seeing patients—two questions for every three patients in one study (Covell, Uman, and

Manning 1985). Give students a chance to choose a question and re-search an answer.

• Use care when questioning students in front of patients. Embarrass-ment will stunt their willingness to expose their reasoning. Questions that clarify their understanding are certainly acceptable—it is the tone and wording that matter most. One approach is to ask questions they likely can answer, particularly early on, thus building confidence. Another technique is to ask questions using graduated success. For in-stance, the teacher can say, "Let's imagine that we are describing this skin lesion to a dermatologist over the phone. Why don't you begin with the size and location?" The student will answer this correctly. The teacher then follows, "Now let's describe its general classification, such as papule, nodule, plaque, blister, or whatever." The teacher lets the stu-dent answer. If the answer is right, the teacher acknowledges this posi-tively. If the student is wrong or unsure, the teacher can say inoffen-sively, "I would describe this as a ——— because ———," thus providing immediate correction.

Enabling Students to Practice with Supervision and Achieve Independence

Practice and repetition are vital for building competence. This is the road to autonomy. The office is both the best and sometimes the hardest place to achieve this. On the one hand, nowhere does the student have a better opportunity to work under one physician's supervision; yet at the same time it can be hard, especially with your own patients, not to jump in and "do things right." Every student and every situation is different. This choice requires supreme judgment. However, it is absolutely necessary to allow students to develop independent clinical skills through practice.

• Set aside visits specifically for supervision. Trainees do far too much clinical work without adequate firsthand supervision—that is to say, they are too often asked to see patients alone, reporting their findings to attendings who then perform their own exams. This does not allow the preceptor to provide feedback based on firsthand observation or to confirm students' ability to perform parts of the history taking or phys-ical exam. Furthermore, practice and repetition without supervision can be counterproductive if mistakes are not corrected.

• Learn to observe without jumping in unless necessary. A helpful approach is to outline before the visit what the student's and teacher's roles will be. For instance, the teacher who wants to observe the student interviewing the patient can say to the student and patient, "I'd like to give Mr. Smith a chance to ask you about your symptoms. Once he completes this—in about ten minutes—I'll ask him a few questions to confirm my understanding, then [to the student] we can meet outside the room to discuss your assessment and plans." Or, "I want to watch you examine the patient's knee so I can see how you do it and give you pointers based on my observation."

Collaborating, Correcting Mistakes, and Demonstrating Competence

Successful teachers create a collegial relationship in which students are not afraid to fail. In this situation students come to expect and welcome honest appraisal, since they are confident about the result—no-fault learning. They know, too, that they will hear when they do well. I will say more about specific evaluation techniques in chapter 8.

• Just as you review goals before each teaching session, review how and when you will correct mistakes.
• Pick a salient point to address; too many corrections will overwhelm a student.
• Ensure that students have an adequate chance to demonstrate important skills. If a skill is worth learning, they should have the opportunity to practice it under supervision. It is important to start at the student's level. Clearly, beginners need more basic instruction than advanced students, but do not be quick to presume that the latter possess sound clinical skills. Many aspects of the history taking and physical exam (e.g., asking an appropriate mix of closed and open questions, performing chest auscultation) have not been adequately supervised during medical school and postgraduate training. Supervised practice in various circumstances is often necessary to detect and correct errors. This is truly one of the great benefits of ambulatory medical teaching. For instance, if a student (even a postgraduate) reports a normal Rhomberg test, it may be important to confirm that it was performed accurately. Rather than simply accepting that the test was done correctly, the pre-

ceptor can say, "When we see this patient together, demonstrate the Rhomberg test." I could cite many examples like this.

Applying Teaching Principles in the Office

Although the ambulatory teaching environment is varied, I envision the reader as a physician working one-on-one with a single medical student or resident in an office setting. The teaching goals and the amount of supervision given naturally differ with the learner and the comfort of the teacher. Also, these techniques and principles can be modified to accommodate other learners (e.g., nurse-practitioner students, medical students working with office staff).

The most common teaching encounters are

1. "Bedside" teaching—the patient, teacher, and learner together
2. "Hallway" teaching—the teacher and learner discussing a problem briefly
3. Minilecture—the teacher and learner in an interactive discussion
4. Chart review—the teacher and student reviewing cases together
5. Planned and unplanned "teaching moments"
6. End of the day "roundup"

Of course this list is not meant to discount other forms of teaching and learning that will occur in the office, such as learning by doing (process learning), interactive computer-based instruction, or informal discussions. It simply organizes the most common teaching encounters you are likely to use in the office.

The tools that are useful in one or more of these settings include

1. Observation, including review of tape recordings or videotapes
2. Asking questions
3. Conscious role modeling
4. Demonstrating skills
5. Keeping a logbook
6. Thinking aloud
7. "Keying in" the learner
8. Researching a problem
9. Role playing

"Bedside" Teaching

The examining room is the most productive setting for teaching and the keystone of the ambulatory teaching experience (Langlois and Thach 2000). Teaching in the patient's presence requires the most skill, since the teacher is monitoring three people at once—the student, the patient, and herself. However, it has many advantages and can be a very rich experience for all three.

The three most common scenarios are these: the student and teacher see the patient together from the beginning of the exam; the teacher comes in midway for part of the exam; and the student asks the teacher to step into the examining room to confirm or consult on a particular issue. These three scenarios tend to follow a gradation from least to most advanced learner, though this is not invariable. Course directors can provide guidance on the readiness and mix of these techniques for different students.

During a patient care visit that is entirely supervised, the attending tries to remain as unobtrusive as possible and watches as the student takes a history and performs an examination. Depending on the clinical situation (i.e., the student sees the physician's patient), the preceptor instructs the patient that he intends to observe without interrupting until the student has completed the examination and then will ask any questions that arise. The teacher should set a time limit. With practice the attending can learn to become a "fly on the wall" and allow conversation to develop between student and patient without excessive interference. If the layout of the examining room permits, the student should be positioned in front of the patient to encourage face-to-face conversation, while the attending stands well to the side. This may seem a little awkward at first, and some patients will tend to turn from the student and direct their answers to the physician. If so, the teacher can gently redirect the interaction by nodding in the student's direction and looking to him for a response. Usually, if the attending focuses on the student during the early phase of the interview, the patient will do this too. Once the interview is under way the conversation between the student and patient will become more natural.

Many visits will be structured so that the preceptor supervises part of the encounter. Typically the attending sets the stage by introducing the student to the patient, followed by some instruction such as, "I'll give Mr.

Jones an opportunity to talk to you, and I'll come back in ten minutes. He can tell me about your problem, and the two of us will examine you together." After this interval the student reports the history—ideally in the patient's presence, but outside the room if need be—then the teacher confirms important elements and examines the patient with the student. This arrangement permits the attending to perform other tasks while the student interviews the patient but still allows some supervision. It is generally preferable to have the student present his findings in the patient's presence. This gives the preceptor more opportunity to see the student interact with the patient, keeps the patient from feeling anxious while waiting alone, and improves the patient's understanding of her medical care. The exception is when a sensitive subject must be discussed out of the patient's presence (e.g., the student suspects surreptitious alcoholism and has not confronted the patient with this concern).

More advanced students (e.g., residents or fellows seeing their own panel of ambulatory patients) often need preceptors to supervise limited parts of the exam or may request only focused consultations (e.g., examine a rash, listen to a murmur). This circumstance may not apply where the attending physician is primarily responsible for the patient's care. Furthermore, it is appropriate that the attending be reimbursed only for work he himself performs and documents. For Medicare this requires that the billing physician observe or perform the evaluation (i.e., history and physical) and contribute to case management for the level that is billed. Program directors can provide guidance for proper documentation.

Except for supervision of advanced learners who follow their own panel of patients or learners seeing patients on return visits, the teacher should ideally review the chart quickly with the learner, which orients the student and increases learning efficiency. In addition, it can focus attention on a piece of information or skill that is worth considering before the student enters the examining room (see "Keying in the Learner" below). For example, the preceptor can say, "Mrs. Jones is fifty-five years old and is coming in because of new back pain. Be aware when you exam her that she was treated for stage 2 breast cancer five years ago. Remember our discussion about 'red flags' when evaluating back pain." This alerts the student to consider dangerous causes for an otherwise common symptom.

You should nearly always set a time limit, convey expectations, and communicate how feedback will be given (see the discussion of the "one-minute observation" below). This need not be elaborate. For instance, "Take fifteen minutes to evaluate this patient with headache. Come get me when you're through and tell me what you think, then we can examine the patient together. I'll go over your notes with you during our break."

The advantages of bedside teaching include

- Providing real-life experience for the student
- Giving an opportunity to model doctor-patient communication
- Observing the student-patient interaction and giving real-time feedback
- Modeling professional behavior
- Demonstrating patient care skills
- Educating the patient and increasing patient satisfaction through participation in the learning experience

Be alert to

- Increasing visit time and schedule delays
- Patient, learner, and staff fatigue

Hallway Teaching

"Hallway" is not to be taken too literally; it refers to teaching done between patient visits—in the physician's office, conference room, library, lab, and such. This is a time for writing notes, answering messages, and communicating with staff. It is also a time for the teacher to give brief, focused feedback on the previous encounter and prepare the student before seeing the next patient.

Excellent teaching opportunities occur during these interludes. Most of the teaching is limited to short questions or remarks, but the student also learns by observing and participating in the office work (process learning). Sometimes the most memorable lessons come from brief comments in the context of the usual work. The preceptor can also use this time to think aloud while performing work (e.g., "I'll give this patient a quick call about her lab while the medical assistant gets the next patient into the examining room. That way we'll have one chart fewer on our stack of messages"). The most important factor to keep in mind is time. When you are teaching it is easy to lose track and answer students with minilectures, but

the main task is patient care, and it is important not to let teaching interfere with this flow. Do not let discussion dominate work or teaching. This
point can be covered with learners during orientation, but it may need to
be reinforced from time to time with a comment such as, "Hold on to that
question and I'll answer it more fully during our break."

Minilectures

The "minilecture" is truly mini, but it is not a lecture—at least not in the
sense of a monologue. It is short, ideally less than twenty minutes and no
more than thirty. A fair characterization would be an interactive discussion between the student and the preceptor. Whether initiated by the
teacher or requested by the student, the best ones are case based. A minilecture can be divided into three sections:

1. The clinical question to be answered
2. The body of the discussion that answers the question
3. The summary, including testing the student's comprehension

Consider a pediatric resident who asks the preceptor to discuss the office-based management of overweight children. The preceptor begins by
referring to a case the two have seen together, a patient she knows, or a
hypothetical case based on her experience. One of them outlines the essential features of the case. To focus the student's attention, the preceptor
asks her to pose a question or questions based on the patient's problem. If
the student has difficulty with this, the preceptor can help. For example,
the student might ask, "What are guidelines for recognizing and treating
overweight children in an ambulatory setting?"

A framework is then developed around the case that includes the question(s) along with a few key points the teacher wants to transmit, such as
defining overweight and obesity, discussing the prevalence and the health
consequences of overweight in children, and outlining the accepted treatment options. The body of the discussion addresses these points. The
teacher gives the student opportunities to supply information or answer
questions from her fund of knowledge, which helps her to stay alert. Also,
questions help the teacher assess the student's knowledge and ensure understanding. Avoid the pitfall of trying to include too much information:
a reference to eating disorders may be appropriate, but discussing how to
treat them would divert attention from the primary question.

As an effective summation, the preceptor might ask the student to reiterate the major points and answer the original question(s) based on the information supplied. An alternative approach might be to pose a hypothetical case and ask the student to evaluate it and propose a treatment plan based on what she has just learned.

These are the important points regarding minilectures:

- Make the discussion case based.
- Begin with a question, preferably one posed by the student.
- Outline a few key points to teach (a blackboard is useful for this).
- Keep the discussion short and on target.
- Use questions to maintain the learner's alertness and ensure comprehension.
- Wrap up by letting the student rehearse and demonstrate the newly acquired information by summarizing the major points and problem solving with a hypothetical case.

Stimulated Chart Review

In stimulated chart review the teacher uses the student's written record of a patient's visit to generate questions that probe the learner's reasoning. The record is used to stimulate the student's recollection of a particular case and recreate his thought process. This technique allows the teacher to review care for one or more patients and helps the student reflect on the decisions he has made. This is particularly useful in clinic situations where residents or fellows have their own panel of patients that are not seen by the attending. It is also useful when an attending physician and a student want to explore in more depth cases seen earlier but do not have time during regularly scheduled clinic visits.

Using the record, the teacher asks the student to recreate the visit, consider the clinical problem, justify the data that are and are not recorded, consider alternative questions that might have been asked, and explain the possible outcomes of therapeutic or diagnostic decisions. Usually you should allow thirty minutes for review and discussion.

For example, a medicine resident reviews the chart of a young woman with diarrhea whom he saw earlier in the day. He describes an eighteen-year-old woman with no previous health problems who has had one day of abdominal cramps with frequent watery stools and one possible sick contact. The patient is not feverish. His record includes a general description of the patient as well as the head, chest, and abdominal exams. He records no observation about volume status in his physical exam and orders a CBC and an electrolyte panel. The attending can begin by asking the resident

1. To describe his first impressions of the patient
2. To state the hypotheses he generated during the encounter
3. To recall what questions he considered when attempting to rule possibilities in or out
4. To list what elements of the physical exam it was essential to perform
5. To justify data included in or omitted from the chart
6. To justify diagnostic and therapeutic decisions
7. To consider alternative approaches to the evaluation and treatment if relevant

Finally, the attending can discuss possible approaches to the problem, keeping in mind that there are often no absolute answers. However, the exercise creates an opportunity for discussion and insight into the learner's patient care decisions in the absence of direct observation.

Teaching Moments

Teaching moments are both planned and unplanned lessons that occur in the course of patient care (Kolb 1985). These discrete experiences have a notable impact on students and are long remembered. Though not all are dramatic events, the impressions they make result from concrete experiences. Later the student is able to reflect on the event and perhaps conceptualize a lesson that can be applied in the future. The teacher can be of great help by providing an opportunity to question and discuss the student's observations. This experience can be described as a cycle, with the concrete experience leading to reflection and observation followed by abstract conceptualization and finally experimentation (Whitman and Magill 2000).

The teacher anticipates planned teaching moments by using clinical experience to foresee memorable events. Often these follow from the natural evolution of patient care. For instance, a preceptor knows that visiting a patient enrolled in home hospice care will give the student an opportunity to learn many important lessons about caring for dying patients. These lessons are best learned by observation and participation. Therefore she invites the student to accompany her on a home visit to the dying patient, preparing him by describing the goals of the visit, which include comforting the patient and family and evaluating the efficacy of pain control. The student is given the role of asking the patient and his spouse about pain control therapy, thus creating a *concrete experience*. In addition, the student makes *observations* about the patient in his environment. The preceptor stimulates *reflection* by asking the student to consider the possible effect of the patient's mood on the efficacy of pain therapy. Later the student and teacher discuss this, and the student draws a lesson about the interaction of mood and pain perception, resulting in *conceptualization* of the experience. The teacher points out other clinical circumstances in which mood affects pain perception and encourages the student to consider this in the future when treating chronic pain. Hopefully the student will test this lesson when seeing other patients with chronic pain (*experimentation*). This begets a cycle that should continue throughout his professional career.

Unplanned experiences abound. The teacher can cue the student, and the student will remember those experiences to the extent that they form an impression. The trick is for the teacher to select and emphasize lessons of value that will be enhanced by reflection. The teacher promotes this by keying the student in to the experience, helping the learner to step back, observe, and later debrief. Take this hypothetical incident. The teacher overlooks a medication interaction when he writes a prescription, and the patient suffers an adverse outcome. The teacher points this out to the student as a lesson to remember and invites him to watch while he explains his mistake to the patient. Later the student is given a chance to discuss his observation and the lesson he learns from the experience.

End of the Day Roundup

Time set aside at the end of the day for communication may be used in any way the preceptor and student feel is important. Generally it is intended to be informal and relaxed. They may simply want to unwind and catch up on loose ends, or they may use the time for feedback and discussion. Often it is helpful to ask the student to cite one new thing learned or relate the most memorable experience for the day. The main point is to provide time, even if it is not explicitly scheduled, for the student to connect with the preceptor and talk about ideas, observations, and the like that seem important.

This informal time may overlap with regularly scheduled evaluative sessions. As rapport builds during a rotation, these sessions become some of the most enjoyable and valuable for both teacher and student.

Observation, Including Videotaped or Tape-Recorded Encounters

In most offices, the teacher directly observes the student-patient interaction. Videotaping or tape-recording is not common (though it may be increasingly feasible as the equipment becomes more affordable). Direct observation allows firsthand knowledge of the student's performance and a chance for immediate feedback (Hinz 1966). Videotaped or tape-recorded sessions offer the advantage of observing more student-patient sessions than would be possible by direct observation alone, freeing the teacher to perform other tasks and to review the student's work at a more convenient time. Another advantage is that they allow students to critique their own performance.

Being observed, and especially being recorded, can be disconcerting for some learners. They should be reassured that stage fright will be discounted and that camera shyness usually diminishes with practice. Still, most students prefer the benefits of direct or indirect observation.

Observation is most fruitful when the preceptor is prepared with a question when watching a student-patient encounter. What do you want to accomplish with the observation? Is it to assess a particular skill and provide feedback? You can note unexpected things too, but preparing a question helps you focus on specific goals. During the office visit, where time is limited and teaching is focused, the "one-minute observation" is an efficient method of providing supervision and feedback (Ferenchick et al. 1997). In this technique the preceptor performs a focused observation of a student-patient encounter, then gives the student immediate feedback. The essential steps are explaining the purpose to the learner and patient; explaining how the observation will be done; making a brief, focused assessment without interrupting the student's exam; leaving the room; and meeting the student for immediate feedback after she completes the exam.

Observation can be aided by either creating a checklist for reference or jotting notes as you watch. A checklist is convenient, produces less distracting commotion, and offers a systematic recording tool, but it can limit notations to those that are predetermined. Scribbling notes can be distracting unless it is kept to a minimum. Also, one may overlook important points if they have not been considered beforehand. Still taking notes allows the preceptor the discretion to record more or less. In either case, if you take notes, you must do it unobtrusively. A useful observation tool is the plus/delta sheet (Qualters 1999), which can be constructed from a three-by-five card. You make two columns: the left side is for what the preceptor likes, and the right side is for what he would like to see changed, including questions for the student. These cards can be ruled to indicate the time flow of the visit so as to provide feedback on efficiency. The cards become a ready reference for feedback and can be saved for later evaluation.

Keying in the Learner

"Keying in" means alerting students to key lessons the teacher wants them to learn. This is similar to a speaker's outlining major points the audience should grasp. With all the activity involved in a patient visit, one cannot assume that students will pay attention to the most salient features. This method is especially helpful when the student "shadows" or observes a preceptor who is interacting with a patient. Keying in can be done before or during a visit.

A student examines a patient whose chief complaint is hip pain. The teacher wants to impress him with the value of having a patient demonstrate an action that reproduces the symptom. He alerts the student by telling him this before he sees the patient. For instance, he can say, "Having a patient demonstrate what causes the problem will often clarify the description of the symptom. Remember to watch the patient getting on and off the exam table, and have him walk for you."

A medical student watches her preceptor check a diabetic patient for sensory loss in the lower extremities. The teacher knows from experience that many students do not explain to patients how they will test for sensory loss, thus confusing them. To draw the student's attention to this, the preceptor tells her, "Before I begin testing for pain sensation, I describe the value of checking sensation and explain how I will do it. Then the patient will understand my questions."

A family practice resident listens as her preceptor explains the result of an echo-cardiogram to his patient. Before beginning the explanation, the preceptor tells the student, "When I'm discussing test results, I'm careful to avoid medical jargon."

Conscious Role Modeling

A teacher is always a role model, for good or bad, consciously or not. Conscious modeling is simply choosing to demonstrate a behavior and keying in the learner beforehand. This can form the basis for later reflection and discussion.

During a busy afternoon a distraught patient stops by to vent his anger because his prescription was not ready when he arrived at the pharmacy. He asks for ten minutes of your time. It is clear that he did not allow enough time for the prescription to be processed. Before meeting with the patient, you brief the student on specifically how you will act addressing the patient and trying to resolve the conflict. You use this opportunity to point out specific values regarding the doctor-patient relationship that you want to demonstrate.

Demonstration

Demonstration is used to teach skills. In the office setting this usually applies to the history and physical exam or to procedures, though it can include behaviors and attitudes in its broadest sense (see "Conscious Role Modeling" above).

There are three elements to consider when teaching a skill (Foley and Smilansky 1980):

1. Analyze the key steps, separate these into component parts, and determine which will be most difficult for the learner to achieve.

2. Model the skill in its entirety; remember to include even basic steps that you take for granted—they may not be obvious to the learner. Modeling may require actual performance, drawings, and oral or written instructions.

3. Supervise the student's practice and ensure mastery.

Demonstration requires the teacher to consider all the steps a task entails. (This includes assembling materials, if any are needed, before the lesson.) The more steps are required, the more preparation is needed (e.g., learning to start an IV). Clearly you must judge the student's readiness to perform any given task and lay the groundwork. You should start at the level of the student; remember that preliminary steps may not be self-evident.

Take the following illustration. A patient is seen in the office for management and evaluation of chronic congestive heart failure. The attending physician wants to demonstrate testing the hepatojugular reflux for the medical resident. To teach this successfully, the preceptor must first consider the steps she is so accustomed to performing:

1. Explaining the procedure to the patient
2. Positioning the patient
3. Identifying the neck veins
4. Measuring the jugular venous pressure
5. Instructing the patient to breathe normally (and avoid Valsalva)
6. Applying steady pressure with the palm over the center of the abdomen (and avoiding direct pressure over the liver)
7. Noting and measuring the response of the jugular pressure

The teacher outlines these steps for the student orally and describes what she is doing while demonstrating each step. After this, she walks the resident through the procedure, including the important preparatory steps, giving feedback and seeing that each step is performed correctly. She also supervises the resident during future patient encounters to ensure competence.

When teaching a student how to improve long-term medication adherence, a preceptor outlines the specific steps she takes. These include setting aside time in the office visit to discuss medications, communicating to the patient her interest in how medications are taken, using open-ended, nonjudgmental questions to determine adherence, problem solving, and reinforcing good adherence behaviors. She has the student refer to a checklist as she demonstrates this skill. She performs these steps during a patient visit and later supervises as the student practices the same steps with other patients until the preceptor is satisfied the skill has been mastered.

Keeping a Logbook

A logbook is a useful tool for students, especially during core rotations. It helps to

- Track individual patients for follow-up
- Review case mix
- Monitor clinical experiences against the learning goals
- Document skills
- Note cases for more detailed discussion
- Generate questions for further research

Thinking Aloud

Teachers can help students gain insight into their thinking by making observations and decisions openly. The idea is simple, but you may need to remind yourself until it becomes a habit. Thinking aloud can take place in the patient's presence or elsewhere.

A preceptor receives a call from a home health nurse regarding a patient she is treating for venous stasis ulcers. The nurse asks for guidance regarding two options: continuing conservative therapy or referring the patient to a plastic surgeon. Rather than weighing the decision silently and giving an answer, the preceptor shares her deliberation with the student. She outlines the steps of her thought process, discussing how she weighs the options and why she chooses one over the other.

While auscultating the heart of a new patient, the preceptor tells him that he hears a murmur and will discuss it with him after he has listened more carefully. To make the process of his exam clear to the student, he says, "I hear a systolic murmur at the left sternal border, and now I want to determine whether it is an ejection or a holosystolic murmur. Holosystolic murmurs begin and end with the first and second heart sounds, and ejection murmurs begin after and end before the first and second heart sounds. I am listening carefully to S1 and S2 to place the murmur in relation to these two sounds."

Role Playing

Both the teacher and the student can role-play. The teacher might use this method to demonstrate a problem, illustrate a point, or provide a lively interaction with the student to test comprehension and problem solving. For example, after examining a patient with peripheral neuropathy, the teacher may want to discuss abnormal gaits. The teacher probably does not have patients who can readily demonstrate these contrasting gaits, but he knows that seeing a variety of gaits will create a more permanent mental image for the student than simply describing them—therefore he acts them out. To impress the student further, he encourages her to follow his lead and act them out too.

In addition to acting for demonstration, the teacher can assume the role of patient, which gives the student practice in interviewing and problem solving. The teacher creates a character, and the student asks the "patient" questions. The teacher controls the answers and can give the student feedback.

For example, the teacher creates a vignette in which he is a forty-year-old construction worker who has been sent by the company nurse for evaluation of high blood pressure. The "patient" is new to the student. He feels fine, he is moderately overweight, and his pressure is 168/95. It is the student's job to take a history, then tell the physician what parts of the physical exam he will perform and how he plans to treat the "patient." The direction of the student's evaluation depends on the answers the teacher gives when playing his role, and the teacher can critique the student's responses.

Research Projects

Research projects during ambulatory rotations typically take two forms: short, focused searches to assist in the management of a specific patient or more expansive research related to best clinical practice. The former is performed almost daily in the context of patient care, the latter over the span of the rotation.

As I noted before, questions are common in everyday practice. Researching real questions that arise in the course of patient care is a necessary clinical skill and a constant feature of lifelong learning. Students should be encouraged to hone this practice using resources available in the office, including Web-based literature searches. This gives them a taste for the challenge practicing physicians encounter and also constitutes a real contribution to the office. Furthermore, students can be encouraged to present this information in the form of a minilecture. In addition to reinforcing their grasp of the material, it gives them experience in teaching.

One final tip regarding research: encourage students to review their patient logs at the end of the day and to identify one problem or question they have. They need not perform an exhaustive search but should simply turn to their favorite text or reference source. Have them read the relevant section, learn a succinct working definition of the disease or syndrome (if appropriate), abstract the important points, and present the information to you at the next opportunity. For instance, the student sees a patient with emphysema. While the experience is still fresh, he learns the definition of the disease, reads about it, abstracts the chapter, and presents the information in ten minutes the next day before seeing patients or during discussion time. This exercise reinforces the student's experience, and the teacher learns something as well.

Summary

• Good clinical teaching in the ambulatory care setting uses principles of adult learning. Effective teachers know their students' needs; identify and organize material that is worthwhile; make information memorable by relating it to immediate problems, experiences, and important concepts; stimulate students to discover and think independently; give students adequate opportunities to practice skills and develop independence; and create a collaborative learning partnership that allows the teacher to correct mistakes and confirm competence.

• In the ambulatory care setting, these principles are applied most frequently in the patient's presence ("bedside" teaching), during interludes between patients ("hallway" teaching), during discussions (mini-lectures), during review of cases (chart reviews), and in teaching moments and end of the day roundup periods. These occasions allow for a balance of direct observation, memorable experiences, discussions, feedback, and informal time between the preceptor and the student.

• Commonly used techniques for teaching in the ambulatory setting involve observation, questioning, role modeling, demonstration, keeping a patient log to record experiences and questions, thinking aloud to reveal problem-solving techniques, keying the learner to salient learning content, researching clinical questions, and role playing.

7

Problems and Challenges in Ambulatory Teaching

Teaching receptive students in an ambulatory setting is immensely satisfying. Yet the challenge of teaching and simultaneously delivering care demands a complex balance of intellectual, physical, and affective skills. The adept clinician who creates the right learning environment and uses the teaching techniques described in chapter 6 will encounter few problems teaching in the office. Still, you may justifiably wonder, "How will teaching in the office affect the flow of patient care, patient and staff satisfaction, and practice income? Furthermore, even in the best teaching programs I'm bound to encounter learners with difficulties. How will I manage this in the office?"

Changes in Office Dynamics

A viable ambulatory medicine practice must provide an environment that is economical and responsive to patients' needs. Timely appointments and a patient-centered staff are absolute requirements. Clinicians who want to teach, usually part time, will have to integrate students into the practice schedule without disrupting the efficient flow of patient services. In this setting, where teaching is a laudable but clearly secondary goal, introducing a learner into the office milieu creates the potential for two problems: disruption in patient care flow and extra demands on staff members' time and focus.

Until you gain experience teaching while seeing patients, the office flow will feel awkward. This rarely persists. The clinician has a great deal of control over the mix of patients students will see and the methods of teaching employed. Furthermore, students, house staff, and other learners invited into an office-based practice appreciate the demands on the clinician's time and want to help, not hinder.

Office staff members often enjoy the interaction with students as much as the teacher does. An eager learner who is interested in operations from the front to the back office will be welcome and will enhance their sense of contributing. Because medical care is inherently unpredictable, they will understand minor disruptions in the routine from time to time; it is the clinician's job to ensure that the staff is given additional time if this is necessary.

If properly prepared, patients generally support teaching (see chapter 4). Many find it confidence building to see their physician trusted to teach. Many enjoy the additional attention of an enthusiastic learner. Some are secret teachers as well. If the clinician reserves private time for those who want it and keeps the schedule moving appropriately, few patients will object to teaching (O'Malley et al. 1997).

Practice income is directly or indirectly dependent on practice flow. Unless they receive a stipend, community-based practitioners will need to maintain their customary patient volume while teaching. Because schedules and clinic responsibilities are so variable, each clinician or practice organization must determine how much time to devote to teaching. For the typical community-based practice, the physician does much teaching while concurrently seeing patients with the student. Practices that can accommodate more advanced learners, such as residents or fellows, may find they can even enhance efficiency (e.g., by seeing unscheduled patients). A workable schedule, as illustrated in chapter 4, usually allows the preceptor to see the same number of patients per session as without a student. If this is done there should be no loss in income. The additional time spent teaching is usually appended to the end of the day. To the extent that teaching is its own reward, practitioners who occasionally teach will find the extra hours spent in teaching or preparation to be the richest form of continuing education.

The following vignette illustrates a clinician's experience while teaching for the first time in the ambulatory setting:

The director for medical education at a nearby medical school asks Dr. Sims, an internist in a busy group practice, to precept medical students in her office. Though she enjoyed teaching as a resident and occasionally supervises medicine house staff when she is attending inpatients, she has no experience teaching in an ambulatory setting. As a preceptor she will supervise one student four afternoons a week during a one-month block of time. She agrees to precept for four blocks a year. Her colleagues, some of whom already precept medical students, are enthusiastic.

Going into her second block, she is having second thoughts about her commitment. On days when she sees patients with a student, she feels rushed, frequently falls behind in the schedule, and leaves the office several hours late. During most patient encounters, the student's evaluations are just too slow for the time allotted. She feels she cannot adequately perform a confirmatory exam, communicate with the patient, and discuss the case with the student. Several patients have been visibly miffed at being kept waiting—and the staff has taken the brunt of this. She wonders if she is just not suited for the pace of ambulatory teaching.

It is unlikely that Dr. Sims is "not suited." She happens to have many skills both as a good clinician and as an effective communicator. Furthermore, she ran her clinic practice smoothly before she introduced students, and she handled multiple patient care tasks deftly. Most likely her inexperience teaching in the ambulatory setting is leading to inefficient time management. Adding teaching to her otherwise busy day clearly requires extra time, but it need not be burdensome.

Dr. Sims examines her experience and consults with a colleague who has experience teaching students and house staff in the office.

She observes that the two medical students have come with similar enthusiasm but different skills and knowledge bases—one has served on an adult medicine inpatient rotation, the other is just starting clinical rotations. Their knowledge, judgment, and physical exam skills seem to be on par with their peers', and they have been open to direction. Both have articulated the same goals: to evaluate and manage common medical problems encountered in an adult ambulatory care clinic, to become proficient in focused exams, to develop outpatient record-keeping skills, and to experience a taste of a clinician's "day."

Dr. Sims's afternoon schedule is divided into fifteen-minute blocks each hour with one thirty-minute block in the middle of the afternoon session for drop-in visits or administrative work. Routine, extended, and new patient visits are allotted fifteen-, thirty-, and sixty-minute appointments, respectively.

Dr. Sims's colleague analyzes the office flow with her and suggests possible problems:

1. Mismatches between students' skill and patient complexity
2. Inadequate preparation of students before patient visits
3. Failure to set time limits on students' workups
4. Failure to save lengthy case discussions for an appropriate time
5. Failure to seize opportunities to work concurrently with students
6. And possibly, scheduling inadequate time for teaching

As discussed in chapter 6, many of these problems will not occur once Dr. Sims learns to implement effective ambulatory teaching skills. Still, losing control of patient flow is disconcerting, and it is easy to forget that a few manageable adjustments can correct the problem.

Matching Students' Skills and Patient Complexity

Preceptors often underestimate the complexity of a learner's task (Westberg and Jason 1993). Even relatively simple problems can pose large hurdles for beginners. When considering students' background and goals, you must match the number and complexity of the tasks to their needs. Those with basic goals need to focus on simple tasks, sometimes just a part of the routine office visit. It is better for learners to concentrate on a few achievable goals than to become mired in many. Later, perhaps on another rotation, they can put all the pieces together.

Preparing Students before Patient Visits

The preceptor often knows the patient. If searching out background information is not the skill the student is learning, then spending time gathering it from the patient or the chart is unproductive. The teacher can assist by supplying context, such as by pointing out past medical information in the chart. The student can thus concentrate on the goal at hand rather than on a tangential task.

Setting Time Limits

Students understand that the preceptor's first priority is to serve the patient. Furthermore, a basic goal in an ambulatory rotation is learning to perform tasks within an appropriate time. Therefore the preceptor should negotiate a time limit for a particular task, then tactfully step in. If you have students' trust, you can unobtrusively signal when you will steer the examination and thereby keep to the schedule. They quickly learn to accommodate.

Saving Lengthy Discussions for Later

Much can be learned if the preceptor explains her thinking as she goes—in other words, thinks out loud. Also, short explanations are often as good as lengthy ones. Questions that require more elaborate answers should be held for breaks or for an end of the day roundup session.

Working Together

Students enjoy contributing as part of a team. For instance, recording a patient's medications or checking blood pressure while the preceptor calls in prescriptions is an acceptable use of their time—especially when the time saved is used for teaching. As far as possible, especially for less advanced learners, the physician should observe and perform patient exams with students. Many tasks can be combined, such as student and patient education or confirming selected parts of the exam while evaluating the learner.

Scheduling Adequate Time

Few practice schedules are designed for teaching, though workable schedules are possible (see chapter 4). The lunch hour and time at the end of the day may be sufficient for minilectures, case discussions, or chart review. In some instances preceptors may need to intersperse office visits with blocks of free time or set aside a few longer visits to accomplish teaching goals. If so, they will need to negotiate an equitable arrangement with the practice or the school. A subsidy or stipend may be necessary.

Using these techniques, Dr. Sims notes steady improvement. She begins to feel less anxious and finds it easier to stay on schedule. Overall, she finds the teaching months pleasurably busy but not overwhelming. Finally the school of medicine agrees to compensate the medical group for one hour of Dr. Sims's time a week. This allows Dr. Sims to expand a fifteen-minute visit to a thirty-minute visit each teaching session, during which she can spend more time observing students with patients.

Managing Problems with Students

Learners who are invited into a community-based practice welcome the respite from the pressures of hospital rotations or even the usual ambulatory clinic affiliated with a teaching hospital. During most ambulatory rotations students and house staff have fewer commitments, time is more structured, and call is less demanding. For many the office practice is a rare opportunity to bask in the one-on-one attention of a clinician committed to teaching. Thus stress and fatigue, factors that commonly account for learning problems or maladaptive behavior, are less likely.

Still, teachers may encounter students whose behavior or interaction with staff interferes with learning or the office environment. Some issues will be specific to the learning situation, but others are more personal and are likely to be problems in other settings as well. What can teachers in the ambulatory setting expect? And how should they respond if a student has problems with learning or behavior?

In general you should expect few serious problems. Most common are correctable difficulties with clinical performance or behaviors the student is unaware of. These are almost always remedied through specific teaching strategies or dialogue. Serious problems with behavior or personality that interfere with performance or staff harmony are uncommon. When these occur you must suspect major deficiencies in training, underlying maladaptation to stress, psychiatric or medical illness, or substance abuse —all requiring attention beyond the ambulatory rotation. You will need to consult the student's program director or dean.

Below is a list of problems taken from my own ambulatory clinical experiences over many years.

Problems of learning or clinical performance include

1. Slow work
2. Poor judgment
3. Knowledge deficiencies
4. Premature closure
5. Vague or noncommittal diagnosis or management

Problems in interacting with the teacher or staff include

1. Argumentiveness
2. Obsequiousness

3. Oversensitivity or defensiveness
4. Excessive interruptions

Problems in interacting with patients include

1. Overinvolvement with patients
2. Unprofessional speech, behavior, or dress
3. Prejudice

Personal problems include

1. Overconfidence
2. Shyness
3. Lack of responsibility, initiative, or motivation
4. Dishonesty
5. Psychiatric illness or substance abuse

Problems of Learning or Clinical Performance

Slow Work

PROBLEM

The learner is forever behind. He cannot meet an agreed-on schedule and does not improve during the rotation. Patients and staff are invariably kept waiting. Rooms and equipment are tied up.

ILLUSTRATION

A medical resident has worked with you four afternoon sessions a week for two months. In spite of his becoming familiar with the patients and office operation, his clinic invariably runs late. His examinations seem inappropriately detailed for the complexity of the problems. Sometimes after completing his write-up or presentation he feels he needs to go back to the patient and check "one more thing."

POSSIBLE CAUSES AND RESPONSES

As discussed above, the teacher can do much to control the pace of closely supervised learners. More advanced learners who do some work independently still benefit from adequate preparation. If the clinician is providing the proper case mix, not overloading the schedule, and not using too much time for case discussions or sign-outs, then these are some possibilities:

• Insecurity about decision making. A learner burned by past mistakes or a harsh teacher may be overly cautious. Discuss the problem and affirm your support and tolerance for mistakes. Teachers can share their own mistakes and what they have learned from the experience.

• Lack of focus or organization. These may represent knowledge deficiencies, inability to set priorities, or occasionally a more general problem in organizing work. Learners who lack knowledge or experience may have difficulty organizing an evaluation or developing a management plan (see "Knowledge Deficiencies" below). Those whose previous experience has been limited to inpatient care will often have an inverted perspective on the urgency and likelihood of problems in the outpatient setting. A short didactic on the most common problems encountered helps. Have learners rank their differential diagnoses from most to least likely and ask them to set priorities for problems. They may need to learn that less urgent problems can be addressed at another visit. Determine whether they have trouble organizing work in other situations. Those who have chronic difficulty in staying organized will need work beyond the limited contact with the preceptor, and you should discuss this with the program director.

• Lack of skill at controlling the pace of the visit. Observing may disclose a problem with interviewing skills (e.g., asking poorly phrased questions that confuse the patient, inadequately mixing open and closed questions, or being unable to control talkative patients). By pinpointing the problem you can make suggestions or demonstrate techniques to quicken the pace.

• Overinvolvement with the patient. See "Overinvolvement with Patients" below.

Poor Judgment

PROBLEM

The student is unable to draw sound inferences from clinical, laboratory, social, and psychological data that balance the potential risks and benefits to the patient. He expresses inappropriate surprise or concern for a problem and alarms the patient.

ILLUSTRATION

A fourth-year medical student sees patients with you in the office during an ambulatory rotation. On a number of occasions he fails to take important symptoms seriously, and at other times he recommends impractical or risky therapeutic plans. He alarms a patient after auscultating the heart by saying, "Wow! That is a loud murmur!"

POSSIBLE CAUSES AND RESPONSES

• Inadequate knowledge or experience. The student may not know the significance of clinical data, may have no experience in implementing therapeutic plans, or may have trouble reading patients' nonverbal messages. Determine whether judgmental errors cluster around a specific skill or knowledge deficiency. If so, you can review the learner's educational experience and make suggestions for strengthening these areas (see "Knowledge Deficiencies" below).

• Fatigue and anxiety. Fatigue and anxiety may impair judgment (Gillis 1993). Although ambulatory rotations are often a respite for learners, some may be balancing academic and extracurricular loads. Use opportunities to discuss possible causes and solutions one-on-one. Refer to the program director if a student's outside responsibilities are too much.

• Difficulty synthesizing medical information. Some learners have chronic difficulty putting all the clinical pieces together. This will likely have been a problem on other rotations and is not easy to solve. Build trust during one-on-one time by sharing experiences, allowing the student to expose his reasoning to constructive analysis. Use open, probing questions ("Tell me your first thoughts when the patient said..." or "What questions could you ask to distinguish between...") to explore his reasoning process (Westberg and Jason 1993). Case discussions, hypothetical cases from your experience, or stimulated chart review can serve as the basis for discussion. In addition, share your own reasoning out loud as you solve problems.

• Alarming patients with inappropriate exclamations or concerns. Bring instances to the learner's attention. Explain the effect on the patient and suggest alternative ways to discuss findings.

Knowledge Deficiencies

PROBLEM

The learner has an inadequate fund of knowledge for the level of training.

ILLUSTRATION

A third-year family practice resident is assigned to work in the office with a surgeon. She appears to be technically skillful and has good knowledge of anatomy. She is deficient in several areas of knowledge that other third-year residents have known. For instance, she does not know the components of the preoperative medical evaluation or the presenting symptoms of common abdominal emergencies.

POSSIBLE CAUSES AND RESPONSES

• Unreasonable expectations by teacher. The teacher may jump to conclusions about a learner's level of knowledge. On a short ambulatory rotation there may be limited opportunity to adequately test competence. Be sure you understand the learner's curriculum, educational experience, and what she is expected to know. If the knowledge base appears to be generally deficient, check the student's past achievement to determine if the current impression is consistent.

• Educational deficiencies. Discuss deficiencies with the learner and determine whether the problem is limited to specific areas (e.g., outpatient evaluation of back pain, therapy for hypertension) or applies to general areas of knowledge (e.g., pathophysiology of pain, principles of drug metabolism). Deficiencies may result from lack of exposure (e.g., missed parts of rotation) or ineffective teaching (e.g., auditory presentations for a visual learner). Specific deficiencies may be remedied by suggesting supplemental reading, lectures, or interactive CDs, by extra skill practice, or by setting aside time for minilectures on the topic. Other techniques: have the student create a presentation on the topic and read a short piece on it each time it comes up. If the problem is a general lack of knowledge, then a comprehensive remedy will need to be implemented through the program director.

• Anxiety. Anxiety may result if the student feels interrogated. Use a nonthreatening tone and posture. Avoid questioning her in anxiety-provoking situations, such as in front of patients or staff. Build confidence by starting with questions the student can answer and acknowledging correct answers (e.g., "Tell me a cause for secondary hypertension. Good! Can you think of any others?" versus "Tell me five causes for secondary hypertension"). Pause after questions; give her time to answer.

• Unclear questions. You may be asking confusing questions. If you are looking for specific information from the student, then ask clear, unambiguous questions. For example, "Describe the fundoscopic findings in open-angle glaucoma" is clear and therefore preferable to "Tell me what you know about the fundoscopic exam in a patient with glaucoma."

Premature Closure

PROBLEM

The student closes a diagnosis before obtaining adequate verification or considering an alternative (Kassirer and Kopelman 1991): in other words, he jumps to conclusions.

ILLUSTRATION

A medical resident jumps quickly from symptom to diagnosis. He often focuses on one feature of a presenting illness or lab value to the exclusion of others and seems to be in a hurry to make diagnoses. When evaluating an older patient with pleuritic chest pain, he ignores the history of sudden dyspnea and relies on chest wall tenderness to confidently diagnose costochondritis instead of the pulmonary embolus the patient has.

POSSIBLE CAUSES AND RESPONSES

• Inadequate hypothesis generation. Deficiencies in knowledge or experience may lead to inadequate hypothesis generation (e.g., if you do not know that acute diabetic neuropathy can mimic a surgical abdomen, it will not be in the differential diagnosis). Strengthening the area of deficiency will help learners broaden their range of hypotheses. Point out strategies for broadening diagnostic possibilities. Use stimulated chart review or cases from your own experience to develop temporal, anatomical, epidemiological, or causal schemes for differential diagnoses. Have learners frame problems before proceeding to the differential diagnosis (e.g., acute large-volume nonbloody diarrhea versus gastroenteritis). This will help them think "general" before getting specific.

• Oversimplification of hypotheses. Students are often taught to find one explanation for a diagnosis ("Occam's razor"), and exclude the possibility of more than one. Old patients or patients with chronic disease may have more than one explanation for symptoms. Students may also think there must be a diagnosis before the patient leaves the office. They may need to learn that sometimes not knowing is acceptable until more information can be obtained.

• Poor interviewing skill. Learners may not have received critical feedback about their interviewing skills and may be unaware of opening the patient interview with leading or closed questions that direct the patient to a narrow response. (*Patient:* "I think I'm getting heart pain." *Student:* "Are you getting chest pain when you exercise?" versus "Can you tell me what you're experiencing?") Use every opportunity to observe learners interviewing patients and bring instances of limiting questions to their attention. Have them practice rephrasing questions using stimulated chart review or role playing.

• Avoiding complicated diagnoses. Overworked or insecure students may unconsciously avoid diagnoses that increase their work burden or expose skill deficiencies (e.g., a student diagnoses gout and plans to treat it with NSAID but fails to consider a septic joint that will require arthrocentesis). Learners may need rest or reassurance, depending on the situation.

• Overconfidence. Some students do not recognize their own limits and rush ahead to a diagnosis before adequately considering differential diagnoses (see the discussion of overconfidence below).

Vague or Noncommittal Diagnosis or Management

PROBLEM

The student is difficult to engage in discussions, uses ambiguous diagnostic terms, or makes vague management recommendations.

ILLUSTRATION

A third-year medical student takes a detailed history and states all the relevant facts about a case. Yet when asked to give his best explanation for the problem he seems afraid to state the obvious. For instance, after examining a seventy-five-year-old woman with one month of morning stiffness, myalgias, and knee joint effusions, he gives as the diagnosis "some sort of rheumatological disease." He eventually tells you the patient probably has polymyalgia rheumatica, but his answers are brief and reveal little about his thought processes.

POSSIBLE CAUSES AND RESPONSES

Lack of precision may cover for a lack of knowledge or fear of giving the wrong answer—particularly if the student has been humiliated for past errors. Using precise language is also a skill that some have simply not developed. In addition to improving communication, precision will help learners think about problems more clearly.

- Lack of knowledge. See "Knowledge Deficiencies" above.
- Insecurity. Give reassurance; keep the atmosphere open for learning. Demonstrate that case discussions are collegial and collaborative—that the teacher and learner benefit from each other's knowledge.
- Poorly developed verbal skills. Have learners summarize case presentations, describe findings, and define terms as precisely as possible. For example: "The patient is a twenty-five-year-old woman with an acute onset of burning pain radiating from the lower back to below the right knee in the L4-5 dermatome" versus "This twenty-five-year-old woman presents with new onset low back pain radiating into the right leg." This exercise helps them solidify their grasp of clinical concepts and develop differential diagnoses. This applies to descriptions of physical findings as well (e.g., "a painful cluster of vesicles on a well-circumscribed, slightly raised red base" instead of "a rash") or definitions (e.g., dysphagia, syncope, congestive heart failure).

Problems in Interacting with the Teacher or Staff

Argumentiveness

PROBLEM

The learner takes a defiant position with the teacher or staff in any discussion.

ILLUSTRATION

The teacher finds himself constantly at odds with an intern working under his supervision. Any suggestion is met with negative statements or arguments. In one instance the intern wants to start an unusually high dose of an antihypertensive for outpatient therapy and the clinician must put his foot down and overrule his decision.

POSSIBLE CAUSES AND RESPONSES

This problem is more common on an inpatient service, where house staff feel a greater sense of "ownership" (Weinholtz and Edwards 1992). For more advanced learners, such as residents or fellows, it may represent a need to demonstrate independence or possibly unresolved anger or stress related to perceived burdens or injustices in responsibilities. Inexperienced learners, such as students, may find the transition from simpler learning governed by rules (e.g., classroom, algorithms for disease management) to more complex clinical judgments difficult and may feel the need to protect their hard-won ground.

- General response. Use diplomatic skills and remain calm; be certain you are not threatening. To determine the cause, open a discussion by stating, "We seem to be disagreeing a lot. Tell me why you think that is." You can respond to argumentive behavior by using active listening, employing I-messages and no-lose negotiations as discussed by Weinholtz and Edwards (1992) and elaborated by Gordon (1977). In active listening, listeners restate the problem in their own words, thereby ensuring comprehension. Use I-messages (e.g., "This is what I have observed," "This is how the problem makes me feel," and "This is the effect the problem is having") to describe the behavior, the listener's reaction to the behavior, and the likely effect of the behavior. No-lose negotiations involve six steps: (1) identifying and defining the problem, (2) generating alternative solutions, (3) evaluating solutions, (4) choosing preferred solutions, (5) implementing the decision, and (6) following up the evaluation. Problems that cannot be resolved should be discussed with the program director or dean.
- Learners want more independence. If an isolated instance does not harm the patient, then be open-minded and respect their independence.

• Difficulty transitioning from simpler to complex clinical setting. Allow students to discuss their frustration. Express empathy and discuss your own experience in making this transition.

Obsequiousness

PROBLEM

The learner pays teacher or staff excessive compliments or uses flattery.

ILLUSTRATION

A third-year student frequently makes comments such as "I can't believe how much you know!" and "You were so on target with that patient—how did you know to ask her that?" She seems too enthusiastic and hangs excessively on the teacher's every word.

POSSIBLE CAUSES AND RESPONSES

Obsequious behavior is recognized by the discomfort it produces in the teacher and staff. Learners who feel vulnerable to evaluation, perhaps owing to past weak performance or lack of knowledge, may behave this way. Occasionally it represents reaction formation when they cannot express hostility to a perceived injustice such as a past unfair evaluation.

• General response. Avoid a negative reaction; a simple formal thank-you will usually signal your lack of interest in trading compliments. If it continues, discuss the problem and determine students' perception of the cause (i.e., unfair evaluations in the past, insecurity about performance).
• Learners feel insecure about evaluation. Review learners' progress; offer assistance to help them achieve course goals and reassure them that fact-based measures will be used to judge performance.

Oversensitivity or Defensiveness

PROBLEM

The learner is unable to accept constructive advice or criticism without making a crestfallen, excuse-filled, or emotional response.

A student offers excuses for every mistake or oversight during his rotation. During an expected midmonth performance review, the teacher uses documented observations to point out deficiencies in record keeping and offer suggestions for improvement. The student appears flustered and blurts out that he has always done things this way and has never been told it was a problem.

POSSIBLE CAUSES AND RESPONSES

If we are honest, even the gentlest criticism is hard to take. We want approval from our mentors. Students are typically vulnerable if they have poor performance and fear failure, are stressed, anxious, or fatigued, or are caught unawares by criticism.

- General response. Open a dialogue. Begin by citing specific examples of the student's difficulty in accepting criticism and ask for his perception of the problem (Sachdeva 1996).
- Giving a critique. Start the critique with reassurance about your motives and acknowledgment of successes. Criticism is easier to digest when it is expected. ("I'll be with you during the interview and give you pointers afterward.") Also, it is best if you can identify with the student as a colleague rather than as an authority. ("I wasn't able to estimate the aortic width reliably until Dr. Smith demonstrated this technique for me. Let me show you what I learned.")

Excessive Interruptions

PROBLEM

The student interrupts discussions with tangential points or questions, interrupts the preceptor's examination of the patient, or interrupts other students and dominates the conversation.

ILLUSTRATION

A teacher is precepting a senior resident and a medical student. During case discussions the teacher cannot complete a thought without the resident's injecting her own. On one occasion when she is observing the preceptor interviewing a patient, she interrupts with her own questions, which are tangential to the preceptor's line of questioning. The teacher is annoyed when, in the middle of a demonstration of the cardiac exam, the resident reaches over to listen with her stethoscope. She also seems to lecture the medical student in an authoritarian tone.

POSSIBLE CAUSES AND RESPONSES

Students who want to impress the preceptor may not appreciate how disruptive their behavior is. Besides being irritating, it can display a lack of decorum to patients, interfere with learning, and destroy team harmony. Learners who are insecure or who want independence will try to demonstrate an authoritative role.

- Student is unaware. Learners, in their exuberance, may be unaware that their approach is inappropriate. Prepare them before you see a patient by outlining the sequence of tasks that the two of you will perform. If you prefer to complete a part of the exam uninterrupted, let them know. If they ask the patient questions at inappropriate times, perhaps while you are palpating the abdomen, step back and tell the patient, "In order to perform this part of the exam properly I'll need to let you relax without speaking." Another tack is to state matter-of-factly, "Let me ask you to save your question until I have finished." If a student is overriding a junior colleague, precede your questions by saying, "This is a good medical student question. Let's see what Jim has to say." The disruptive student will get the point.
- Students want to demonstrate knowledge, independence, or leadership. Give them opportunities to give minilectures, lead case discussions, or demonstrate skills.

Problems in Interacting with Patients

Overinvolvement with Patients

PROBLEM

The student becomes overly bound to patients' care and outcomes and may see herself as responsible for every aspect of care.

ILLUSTRATION

A nursing student complains of fatigue and inability to get work done. She is taking longer than necessary with her patients, often working out details of care that could be done by others. She feels guilty when a patient's outcome is not perfect and takes personal responsibility.

POSSIBLE CAUSES AND RESPONSES

Students may have difficulty determining their professional boundaries (Duckworth, Kahn, and Gutheil 1994). They may find it hard to trust enough to delegate work, have an unmet personal need (e.g., permission to take time off), or feel that approval is related to the amount of time they spend with patients. Discuss the problem to determine the cause.

- Inability to delegate work. Discuss what professional roles it is appropriate to delegate, including ways to sanction and record that responsibility. Students may benefit by spending time with office personnel to learn about their responsibilities. Use case discussions or role playing to demonstrate points.
- Unmet personal needs. Talk to students and help them see healthier long-term ways to meet their needs.
- Associating extent of patient involvement with good care. Demonstrate how you successfully manage patients by using your time efficiently. Use one-on-one time to discuss outside interests, how to balance social and professional life, and so on. Be certain you are not signaling the opposite message by your own actions or rewarding excessive work.

Unprofessional Speech, Behavior, or Dress

PROBLEM

The student's unprofessional speech, behavior, or manner of dress is interfering with the clinician-patient relationship.

ILLUSTRATION

A medical student comes to a geriatric outpatient clinic dressed in an open-necked polo shirt and tennis shoes. He is not wearing his name tag. In front of the patient he presents while leaning back with his foot against the examining room wall. Several patients voice their disapproval and ask if medical schools are no longer teaching professional decorum.

Although schools may attempt to set professional standards for dress and behavior, general culture has changed, and students may not hear this message clearly. Occasionally their demeanor represents a form of attention getting, though more typically it is a simple lack of training. Appropriate dress and grooming may differ depending on the setting. Proper identification is particularly important to patients (Menahem and Shvartzman 1998).

• Lack of awareness or training. Discuss symbolism of clothing, grooming, and speech (e.g., patient introductions, norms for using formal and informal names) and demonstrate by good role modeling. Assign reading or discuss factors that influence the clinician-patient relationship.

Prejudice

PROBLEM

The student forms opinions about patients based on group affiliations that interfere with communication or care management decisions.

ILLUSTRATION

A physician's assistant student, who was once obese, is an exercise enthusiast. He seems to take an inflexible position with obese patients and often has little patience if they are not interested in weight loss. He expresses the opinion that these people are lazy and weak willed and tends to spend less time with them. A discussion reveals his own fear of becoming obese again.

POSSIBLE CAUSES AND RESPONSES

Although overt expression has become less common, prejudice may still be held covertly or unconsciously. Prejudiced beliefs may be learned or may be defensive reactions to fears projected onto a certain group. Prejudiced behavior may become apparent if the learner avoids certain groups (e.g., gay patients out of fear of HIV infection), expresses unjustified beliefs (e.g., obese patients are unhappy with their self-image), or presumes values when making management decisions (e.g., old patients do not want aggressive medical therapy).

• General response. Cite specific examples and explain the possible effect on the patients' care. Discuss professional ethics and responsibility to patients. Suggest literature that may provide access to patients' values and improve the learner's self-knowledge and understanding of the clinician-patient relationship (Hunter, Charon, and Coulehan 1995).

Personal Problems

Overconfidence

PROBLEM

The learner acts more advanced than his level of experience warrants.

ILLUSTRATION

A medical student resists waiting for the teacher to confirm management plans before discussing these plans with patients. He uses phrases such as "in my experience" when this is clearly inappropriate. He speaks to patients in an authoritarian or patronizing tone.

POSSIBLE CAUSES AND RESPONSES

Learners who display this characteristic may be self-absorbed, believing their own message, or may simply be reacting to insecurity. In either case you should discuss your concern with them and be vigilant for the patients' safety.

• Self-absorption. The learner may have a personality trait that you are not likely to influence on the rotation. Consult the program director or the student's dean.
• Insecurity. Spend time discussing the limits of medical certainty and the pitfalls of being too self-assured (e.g., losing the patient's confidence when a diagnosis or treatment is different than expected). Demonstrate collaborative behavior with patients and colleagues. Discuss how this augments communication and improves patients' adherence to medical care. Be certain you are not using authoritarian communication (speech or body language).

Shyness

PROBLEM

The learner is excessively reserved and has difficulty forming warm, friendly relationships with patients and staff.

ILLUSTRATION

A medical resident from England is respected for his clinical acumen and good judgment, but he has little interaction with office staff and does not join in the usual office small talk. He comes across as formal during presentations and case discussions yet seems genuinely caring with his patients.

POSSIBLE CAUSES AND RESPONSES

The reserved learner may be shy by nature, may be anxious about forming relationships, or may be conforming to a personal or cultural norm. It is a problem if it interferes with effectiveness with colleagues, staff, and patients.

- Shy personality or anxiety. Minor shyness or anxiety in new relationships can usually be overcome by establishing a warm atmosphere and inviting learners to join informal gatherings of staff (e.g., lunchtime). If it is more severe, then discussion with students and the program director or dean is necessary in order to implement therapy.
- Personal or cultural norm. Model and discuss with students how you respond to patient and staff needs for communication and social interaction. Discuss how behavior that may seem spontaneous is sometimes intended to create an atmosphere or effect.

Lack of Responsibility, Initiative, or Motivation

PROBLEM

The learner cannot be counted on to perform work reliably. He seems uninterested and exhibits little initiative for doing more than the minimum necessary.

A senior medical student who is interested in surgery is assigned to your practice during part of a medicine rotation. On more than one occasion he shows little interest in participating in roundup discussions of medical management at the end of the day. He is content to follow you around and has no desire to see patients on his own. He shows up late on several occasions and calls in once to cancel because he does not want to miss a surgery conference.

POSSIBLE CAUSES AND RESPONSES

Students see some aspects of medicine as inherently more interesting than others. Consequently they may not appreciate what they can learn from different disciplines. Some may be genuinely fatigued from overwork.

   • Irresponsibility. Discuss the work ethic. Insist on reasonable work responsibilities that must be met.
   • Lack of interest. Review students' goals. There may be aspects of the office's operation that they can appropriately spend more time on. Alternatively, they may accept a research project that unites their interest with the practice (e.g., use of compressive dressings for outpatient treatment of stasis ulcers).

Dishonesty

PROBLEM

The student shows a lack of honesty when demonstrating knowledge. She claims to have performed parts of the exam that were not done. She is not truthful about fulfilling responsibilities.

ILLUSTRATION

A medical student interprets a physical finding erroneously and claims it was taught to her in this way. On another occasion she states that a patient denied having a black, tarry stool when it is clear that she did not ask. She misquotes lab results and later says this is what she remembered. She misses clinic, suggesting that she is sick when in fact she is not.

POSSIBLE CAUSES AND RESPONSES

Though some students who lie lack a well-developed sense of right and wrong, lying is often a maladaptive defense to a perceived need for perfection. Teachers may inadvertently promote dishonesty if they create unreasonable expectations for work or knowledge.

- Maladaptation to stress. Discuss the value of integrity. Explore the possible causes, such as a fear of not knowing everything or past experience of harsh criticism for wrong responses. Reassure learners that you value integrity over knowledge.

Psychiatric Illness or Substance Abuse

PROBLEM

The student exhibits serious emotional or behavioral problems during the rotation that preclude patient care.

ILLUSTRATION

A psychiatry resident often appears distracted at work. She shows little interest in her patients and has missed clinic several times because of illness. She delivered a healthy full-term baby nine months earlier and worries incessantly about the child's safety in day care. One day she bursts into tears and remains inconsolable. She has to leave for the rest of the day. You notify the program director, who arranges for her to have a medical examination. Later the resident calls to thank you for your help and tells you that hypothyroidism was diagnosed. She is on thyroid replacement hormone and is feeling well again.

POSSIBLE CAUSES AND RESPONSES

The preceptor's response to seriously impaired students should be limited to support and reassurance that strict confidentiality will be maintained, while referring them to the program director's or dean's office. As this case illustrates, behavioral problems may not be what they seem, and as in all circumstances a thorough evaluation is necessary before conclusions are drawn; it is beyond the preceptor's role to attempt more than helping students get appropriate assistance.

Summary

• Preceptors in the ambulatory medical setting can do much to provide a supportive, collegial learning environment.

• Clinicians who host medical students or residents in the office can expect the vast majority to be receptive learners who are eager to contribute to the smooth flow of the office operation.

• When teaching slows the work flow, the preceptor can usually correct the problem. This is accomplished by matching students' skill to the complexity of the task (e.g., novices with simple tasks, advanced students with more complex tasks); preparing students before seeing patients; setting workable, firm time limits on students' tasks; postponing lengthy case discussions until an appropriate time; having students perform some tasks independent of the preceptor; and allowing adequate time in the schedule for supervision and teaching.

• Most problems with learners are not serious. When you do encounter problems, the following steps are generally successful: address problems promptly and directly; use specific examples; maintain an open, problem-solving dialogue with learners; monitor improvement and give feedback; and consult with the program director or dean about recurrent or serious problems outside the scope of the brief ambulatory rotation.

8

Evaluating the Learner and the Teacher

One month after precepting in his office, a physician reviews the student's evaluation of his teaching. He is a bit surprised by the report. It is clear that the student was caught off guard by the preceptor's written comments indicating that he performed generally well but needed to strengthen a few specific areas. The teacher thought he had communicated this during the rotation, yet the student reported that he did not receive adequate feedback to correct the deficiencies noted in his evaluation. The preceptor recognizes that in the future he must prepare learners to receive feedback and be clearer when he is providing it. He decides he will ask the program director about resources that will help him improve this aspect of teaching.

Dr. Jones was once apprehensive about providing feedback to students, especially correction. She feared that criticizing their performance would spoil her rapport with them. However, her own experience in receiving feedback from her colleagues has taught her that, when well done, even corrective feedback is appreciated. Furthermore, she sees that evaluation and feedback help her students progress toward their learning goals more efficiently. She is convinced that feedback is as important to her educational mission as the content of her instruction. Now, at the beginning of every rotation she sets the stage by creating a collaborative learning environment in which her students look forward to her observations about their performance. They respect her medical judgment and trust that her critique is designed to enhance their professional growth. Furthermore, they feel free to tell her what helps them most. In their course evaluations, many comment that they wish more attendings would provide corrective feedback in the way Dr. Jones does.

At the beginning of each learning session Dr. Smith asks students to identify a specific goal they want to concentrate on. Sometimes she suggests goals based on her knowledge of their needs. To help them meet their goals, she has learned

from experience to inform students explicitly that she will evaluate their performance and give feedback based on her observation and that the sole purpose is to
help them become successful. She reassures them that at no time will they be embarrassed in front of patients or staff. In addition to giving feedback during or immediately following patient encounters, she makes sure she schedules frequent
informal feedback sessions during the rotation. She uses these times to discuss
their performance on specific tasks. She also schedules a midrotation meeting to
review general progress and give a formal evaluation. She freely asks students to
give her feedback too. She wants to meet their needs and often asks, "Is there
something I can do differently to help you reach your goals?"

During evaluation preceptors analyze students' performance, report
their observations to them, and then encourage them to stay on course or
else help them correct mistakes. Such evaluation is essential for learning
and implicit in everything I have written to this point. Without evaluation, which includes assessment and subsequent feedback, students are
left adrift, which can create anxiety. Where do they stand in relation to
their goals? This is particularly true for novices learning clinical medicine, a field characterized by complexity, uncertainty, and ambiguity
(Gruppen 1997). Motivated learners thus seek evaluation and look for
ways to improve their performance even when explicit direction is lacking—whether by gleaning hints from preceptors' expressions or by studying the outcome of their own decisions. Yet in spite of the crucial role
evaluation plays in the development of clinical skills, it is too often missing or delivered ineffectively. When it is not missing altogether, it is often
too general, based on secondhand reports, or untimely and distant from
learners' experience. Therefore it is easy to understand students' frustration when teachers do not provide clear feedback (Irby 1986).

Consider the student's challenge when evaluation is lacking. The
teacher directs her to meet a goal, one that is often complex and ambiguous (e.g., "Complete a focused exam of this patient with chest pain").
She performs the task to the best of her ability, yet the accuracy and com-
pleteness of the exam are not self-evident. In spite of this, the teacher fails
to come behind her and say straightforwardly, "You performed these components of the exam but omitted these. These parts you did well, and

these will need further work." How does she proceed? In a word—blindly. At this point, without clear coaching, the student must grope for hints of success or failure. She is left to her own wits and must divine clues, verbal or nonverbal, from the preceptor or others. Unfortunately these clues are not always reliable, and thus she runs the danger of perpetuating and reinforcing mistakes. Likewise, the learner cannot be faulted for assuming that no news is good news—even though this may foster a misunderstanding. What if she believes her performance is better than it actually is? And even if the student performs the assignment well, without a timely, accurate report from the teacher her learning is not as efficient as it could be—to say nothing of her worrying about her progress.

Clinical teaching need not suffer this way, especially when there is a solid one-on-one relationship between preceptor and student. In the ambulatory setting, where the two develop a collaborative learning partnership, evaluation should be expected and welcomed (Sachdeva 1996). If the teacher and student discuss how evaluation will be conducted and set times to discuss performance, then it will flow naturally from their dialogue. In this context it becomes a regular habit, remains helpful, and lacks the negative connotations associated with criticism or judgment. It becomes a valued, anticipated component of problem solving and a learning tool they share (Quattlebaum 1996).

So what characteristics make evaluation optimally effective? On the following points teachers and students agree. It should be sufficient, timely, regular, and relevant. In addition, it should provide encouragement, make specific recommendations for improvement, and allow the student to reciprocate by giving feedback to the teacher (Hageman 1988; Sachdeva 1996).

Evaluation encompasses both an assessment of the student's performance and feedback about results. In this context assessment and feedback are part of the same cloth. To provide effective evaluation, the teacher must consider the following:

1. The purpose of the evaluation: to inform the student and others of his progress and achievement, correct mistakes, reinforce good performance, and motivate

2. The source of the student's evaluation: self, teacher, and patients

3. How and when to deliver the message
4. Follow-up and reinforcement of the message
5. Reciprocal feedback from the student

The Purpose of the Evaluation

Evaluation serves four important functions:

1. To assess the student's performance and inform him and others (e.g., program director) of his achievement relative to the course goals
2. To help the student reach those goals by correcting mistakes
3. To motivate
4. To reinforce good performance

The ultimate purpose of evaluation is to help the student. Of course program directors want to know how well students perform. They need to know how ably they meet the course objectives and may use preceptors' assessments to rank them in relation to their peers. But the teacher's first responsibility is to the student. To meet this responsibility she provides the student with clear and consistent information about performance. This requires that the preceptor measure the student's progress and point him along a suitable course. When the preceptor sees good practice, she strengthens it. The teacher also motivates the student to do well. Putting evaluation in the context of helping eliminates much of the anxious fretting about hurting teacher-student rapport, harming the student's self-esteem, or creating a confrontation. The student wants help, and the preceptor is there to give it. Still, good intentions are not a formula for effectiveness. But if the teacher starts with the premise that evaluation is primarily to serve the learner, much of what follows will be easy to implement.

Based on an assessment of the student's performance, the preceptor gives feedback. Feedback provides the student with knowledge of results, validating the student's own impressions about his performance. It can be informational or motivational.

Informational Feedback

Informational feedback addresses learning content and assesses learning needs within the domains of knowledge, skills, and attitudes. It reports students' achievement and gives them concrete guidance. Where they fall short of learning goals, informational feedback increases their awareness of their performance and provides additional instruction on how to improve. If the deficiency is knowledge based, then teachers identify the specific knowledge content students lack, suggest informational resources, and outline a study plan. For example, a student who cannot distinguish among common forms of vaginitis may be assigned supplemental reading to be reviewed with the teacher. Similarly, once a skill deficiency is recognized and discussed, the teacher needs to make provisions for increased supervision and practice of that particular skill. As I noted earlier, attitudinal behaviors are difficult to teach, and they are also hard to correct. However, a crucial step is providing the informational feedback to help students recognize the problem. Once the behavior is clearly defined, you should engage in a dialogue, enabling the student to gain insight into the undesirable behavior and to consider acceptable alternatives. Students actively model the behavior of their mentors. You can provide additional informational feedback by modeling the preferred behavior and pointing out what you are doing.

Motivational Feedback

Motivational feedback is based on an overall evaluation of performance. For instance, is the student developing the skills of a self-directed learner? Does she need a gentle push to increase confidence? Will she benefit from general encouragement to stay the course? Depending on students' behavior, preceptors may use incentives or deterrents to direct them along the desired path. Internally motivated students may respond to opportunities for greater autonomy and achieve satisfaction from accomplishing the task. Those that are externally motivated may respond better to rewards such as grades or promotion. Positive feedback itself is motivational. Negative feedback may be motivational too, unless it is embarrassing or perceived as punitive, in which case it may harm students' confidence and growth.

Reinforcing Good Practice

Feedback should be used to reinforce good performance and desirable behaviors (Opila 1997; Borum 1997). Positive feedback is most effective for this. Considering its power, it is unfortunate that it is used so little in clinical teaching. Once a student demonstrates good practice, the teacher should acknowledge it positively. This is the surest way to see that desired behavior will be repeated and sustained. Take a preceptor who coaches students to stop patients periodically and summarize their history to ensure understanding. When she observes students practicing this technique during a patient's exam, she can reinforce it by specifically acknowledging the behavior. A statement such as "I noticed that you periodically stopped to summarize the patient's history in your own words and asked her to confirm your understanding; that's a good way to ensure the accuracy of your history" gives students clear information about what they have done well and increases the chance that they will continue to do it. Not only do these positive messages reinforce and sustain good performance, they also improve acceptance of corrective feedback when it is necessary.

The Source of the Evaluation

When students are uncertain of their skills, they rely chiefly on external sources of evaluation. In the ambulatory setting the primary source for evaluation is the preceptor, but other sources include self-appraisal, outcomes from tasks, and feedback from patients. As students gain experience and confidence in their skills, they will rely increasingly on self-appraisal and task-related outcomes. This is a long-term goal for self-directed learners—to develop a true sense of their skills and the ability to judge their own performance. Each source has potential value and provides a useful perspective, but teachers are ultimately responsible for evaluating performance. Thus they must ensure that students receive maximally effective feedback.

Credibility and Trustworthiness of the Source

To be maximally effective in changing behavior, the feedback source must be credible and trustworthy. Credibility depends on students' perception of their teachers' expertise; trustworthiness depends on perception of their motives. Therefore, teachers who are seen as knowledgeable, who use clinical skills effectively, and who encourage students to succeed are credible and trustworthy and are in the best position to influence behavior. This is particularly true when students work in an unfamiliar setting or face an unfamiliar task. In these circumstances they are most likely to look to external sources for feedback. Later, as they gain experience, they become more confident and look to their own performance to judge competence. Thus, early on students rely mainly on their teachers for feedback, whereas advanced learners depend more on self-appraisal and on the task itself. For advanced learners preceptors must find a balance between giving feedback often enough to keep them on track and reinforce good practice and not wresting away their sense of internal control.

Consistency of Feedback from Different Sources

Because feedback comes from various sources, teachers must ensure that it is consistent. Consistent feedback reinforces the intended message and is perceived as more accurate. Inconsistent feedback creates anxiety and may convey the wrong message. For example, when the student receives feedback from the teacher and the task simultaneously, the two sources may seem to conflict. When this happens the teacher must help the student reconcile the disparity. If there is inconsistency between the task-related performance and the teacher's feedback (e.g., student arrives at the correct diagnosis yet teacher faults the reasoning that leads to the diagnosis), the student will likely downplay the importance of the teacher's unfavorable feedback in favor of the positive task-related feedback. Positive feedback (in this case, correct diagnosis) is generally favored over negative feedback (incorrect reasoning), regardless of the source. Positive feedback will be overvalued and negative feedback discounted. The teacher should recognize the potential for feedback disparity and bring it to the student's attention. For instance, he might say, "Even though your diagnosis is correct, the steps you used to reach it were deficient for these reasons. By omitting the following steps you could miss important alternative diagnoses. Let me illustrate what I mean." The teacher acknowledges both messages and helps the student make sense out of the apparent contradiction between the results and the process used to achieve them. If the teacher simply comments on the faulty reasoning, the student may give less credence to the feedback. Furthermore students who remain uncertain why the discrepant messages coexist may leave the encounter feeling anxious because they lack any sense of inner control to evaluate their own performance.

Positive feedback from the teacher, on the other hand, will be preferred over negative feedback from the task, since positive feedback is more readily accepted. Teachers should be especially cognizant of this tendency when giving positive feedback if other sources are giving important negative messages that learners must recognize. What if the teacher chooses to praise the student for charting preventive health measures during a patient's office visit yet the learner feels overwhelmed by the number of tasks required during a routine visit? The student may be anxious about the conflicting messages yet may not say so. The teacher may have to infer this from behavior, expression, or body language. Once the conflict is recognized, the teacher can address the anxiety by acknowledging both messages—that charting preventive health care is desirable and also that one may feel overwhelmed by too many tasks. This positively acknowledges the desirable behavior and helps the student respond by learning to budget time effectively. The teacher acknowledges the task-related negative feedback and puts it into perspective.

Self-Appraisal

In addition to seeking external sources of evaluation, students should be encouraged to appraise their own performance. After they attempt a task, teachers should ask them for their own views of what does and does not work. This is particularly helpful before teachers initiate a discussion during a feedback session and will help them understand students' perspective. However, self-appraisal alone is not sufficient; it should be linked to a discussion with the teacher. Self-appraisal and subsequent discussion increase students' perception of the feedback's accuracy and improve its acceptance. Furthermore, without discussion and guidance, students may misinterpret task-related feedback or miss the important features of their performance. Also let me stress that self-appraisal without discussion is not satisfying for novices. Dialogue about performance that incorporates students' self-assessment yields greater satisfaction with the feedback and greater motivation to change.

Feedback from Patients

Patients, too, are a valuable and unique source of feedback. By seeking their perceptions and intuitive comments, students can gain an appreciation of patients' feelings and the impact they have on their health care. Furthermore, patients do not seem to be intimidated by offering feedback. Most are flattered, and contributing in this way increases their participation in the teaching endeavor (Falvo 1980).

It is not uncommon for patients to give to students positive but general feedback. Preceptors can help patients provide specific comments on students' performance. A patient may remark, "I believe Mr. Jones will make a good doctor." The reflexive response might be to say "I agree." Yet the teacher can plumb the remark a little deeper by asking, in the student's presence, "What did you like most about your visit with Mr. Jones?" An answer such as "I liked the way he listened; he let me talk about my problems even though I know there aren't easy solutions" gives the student firsthand information—and a lesson he won't likely forget—about what the patient valued most. Without the patient's input, this kind of feedback can only be inferred.

In addition to spontaneous comments, preceptors can obtain information from patients by using a systematic format (Tamblyn et al. 1994). The receptionist can distribute a short postvisit questionnaire, to be reviewed during evaluation sessions. Ideally it should be combined with direct observation. Without direct observation the preceptor may not be able to help the student correct behavior. If direct observation is not always feasible, the survey at least serves as another perspective on performance and can be valuable in spite of this limitation.

How and When to Deliver the Message
Timely, Objective, and Specific Evaluations

Evaluations should be timely, objective, and specific and should be delivered in a way that promotes maximum acceptance. To accomplish this, feedback should be given as close as possible to the activity being evaluated. It should be based on facts, preferably those that are observed directly. Feedback should be worded clearly so the learner understands precisely what action or behavior the teacher is evaluating. And finally, it should be offered constructively so the student is not threatened.

Students commonly complain that clinical teachers give too little feedback too late. Teachers can remedy this by preparing students to receive regular feedback, by giving feedback during clinical supervision (formative feedback), and by scheduling evaluative sessions to review progress and achievement in the middle of a rotation and again at the end (summative feedback). Generally speaking, formative feedback and performance assessments are easier to deliver and accept when students are prepared to hear them. Building regularly scheduled sessions into the rotation and negotiating how feedback will be given helps them prepare mentally so they do not feel blindsided by a process that may initially seem intimidating.

Preparation for feedback begins at the start of the rotation and should be part of the learning contract. Students should also be briefly reminded at the beginning of each learning session of how and when feedback will be given.

During the orientation session the teacher lays out the framework for feedback. This includes the timing and the way messages are given. For example, the student may be told that feedback will occur during or immediately following each learning session and that he will be free to make comments and ask questions. The teacher also indicates that she will ask the student for suggestions about her teaching style and content as well.

Some students will see only formal evaluative sessions as feedback. They may fail to recognize feedback that is concurrent with teaching (and complain that they did not receive it) unless it is explicitly identified as feedback from the teacher. Therefore teachers should state before each teaching session and at the time feedback is being given that comments on performance are indeed feedback. In fact, until students are accustomed to receiving feedback, it is wise to make a habit of saying, "Let me give you some feedback," before making comments on performance. In this way there is little chance of misunderstanding the teacher's intent.

Formative Feedback

Formative feedback is given in the course of daily practice, as close as possible to actual performance, when memory of details is freshest. At this time feedback has the greatest influence on specific behavior. Feedback that is even a day old is not as helpful and has less chance of motivating a change or reinforcing a desired behavior. Of course, the precise timing depends on the circumstances. Positive feedback is easiest to give immediately. Negative feedback should be given as soon as possible too, but it may need to be postponed if it risks embarrassing the student or damaging the patient's esteem for the student or if it comes at an emotionally charged moment. However, corrective feedback is usually well accepted if the student is prepared to hear it and it is delivered properly.

In some cases it is necessary to give corrective (though not harsh) feedback in the patient's presence—for instance, when a preceptor supervises a student during a procedure or physical exam. Feedback need not embarrass the student as long as it is worded tactfully and the student is prepared for the teacher's comments. A statement helps forecast the teacher's intent. For example, if the preceptor says to the student, "I'll offer feedback as we go along," neither the student nor the patient is surprised by tactful guidance.

It is not always necessary to give feedback during or even immediately after a patient visit. Teachers cannot sacrifice efficient patient flow or patients' needs to provide all the feedback necessary. Also, they may not want to overload students. Brief comments on performance, leaving time for discussion later, are entirely appropriate. Preceptors who feel that feedback should be postponed until later in the day can say so. They may comment quickly that they would like to give the student feedback but, owing to time constraints, will postpone it until a predetermined time—perhaps a break in the clinic schedule or at the end of the day. The timing can be arranged at the beginning of the learning session so students know they will have an opportunity to discuss their performance. For example, a preceptor may watch a student perform an entire physical exam yet not have time to comment on all of her observations. She may use a checklist or a brief note to help her remember important observations she wants to discuss later. After the exam, she says, "I have few suggestions that will improve the following parts of your physical exam. Remind me to discuss these during our break together at lunch."

Summative Evaluations

Summative evaluations give students an overall report on performance, allowing them to assess their accomplishments in relation to the learning objectives for the course and their peers' performance. Summative evaluations are typically formal, and the learning contract serves as a reference. The results may be oral or written. When evaluations are written, however, they should not substitute for a discussion with the student unless there are extenuating circumstances.

A summative evaluation looks at trends in performance over time. As such it takes a broad perspective, pointing to a direction the student is taking in various areas of competence and behavior. Summative evaluations for ambulatory rotations typically encompass the following general areas:

1. Knowledge (understands important principles, knows relevant medical information and literature)
2. History and physical skills (uses skills efficiently and appropriately, focuses skills appropriately)
3. Procedure skills (competence, appropriateness)
4. Effectiveness of patient care (develops workable, cost-effective care plans)
5. Independent learning (reads, uses reference sources, researches problems, uses evidence-based principles)
6. Record keeping (keeps high-quality notes, charts information appropriately, documents patient encounter or care, writes legibly)
7. Communication (communicates concisely with colleagues, communicates effectively with patients and staff, offers effective patient education)
8. Clinical reasoning and judgment (makes logical diagnosis, uses tests or lab work sensibly, integrates information into workable care plans)
9. Approach to emergencies or urgent illness (recognizes them and responds appropriately)
10. Responsibility, initiative, and motivation (can be relied on, shows enthusiasm)
11. Work efficiency (exhibits promptness, organization, and good use of time)
12. Rapport with patients and families
13. Humaneness of patient care
14. Relations with office staff
15. Professionalism

These general skills and attributes are organized to reflect specific objectives for a curriculum. An example is taken from the Johns Hopkins General Internal Medicine Residency Program Community-Based Practice Evaluation Form (table 8.1).

It is readily apparent that the evaluation should serve as a tool for the learning contract. Preceptors should review the form (or at least its major

Table 8.1. Johns Hopkins General Internal Medicine Residency Program Community-Based Practice Evaluation Form

Clinical care: quality

Uses evidence-based approach to clinical decision making

Aware of risk/benefit, interactions, adverse reactions in prescribing medications

Reliably follows up tests, consults, interval care

Prioritizes problems appropriately

Recognizes acute illness, emergencies, "can't miss" diagnoses

Knowledgeable in related areas (Gyn, Derm, Ortho, ENT, Ophtho)

Implements appropriate preventive interventions

Performs accurate physical examinations

Establishes sensible differential diagnoses

Familiar with approaches to common primary care conditions

Probes for and recognizes mental illness and substance abuse

Counsels patients effectively

Clinical care: utilization

Uses diagnostic tests judiciously and appropriately

Refers judiciously and appropriately to consultants/others

Uses case managers/home health services appropriately

Spends time with patients appropriate to complexity

Focuses history and limits exam appropriately

Prescribes medications cost effectively, using formularies as indicated

Doctor-patient relations

Ensures accessibility to patients by phone or appointment

Makes an effort to see patients on time or explains waiting period

Communicates courteously and effectively with patients

Addresses patients' beliefs, feelings, expectations, concerns

Effectively uses patient education and behavioral change strategies

Manages complaints/anger/demands of patients sensitively and effectively

Demonstrates empathy and compassion for patients

Assesses family and social context of patients' illnesses and behaviors

Deals effectively with family concerns

Manages phone calls in a timely, courteous, and effective manner

Reliably communicates diagnostic test results to patients

Attends to patient dignity and comfort in examining room

Table 8.1. (continued)

Professionalism, staff relations, teamwork

Respects and works well with support staff

Adheres to practice policies and procedures

Contributes to changes and improvements in practice

Is punctual

Is mindful of appearance and professional demeanor

Documentation, billing, productivity

Maintains medical records according to standards

Makes visit notes that accurately and efficiently reflect patient encounters

Codes/bills appropriately

Is efficient and productive in seeing patients

Self-directed learning

Assesses and communicates own learning needs

Independently reads or seeks out information relevant to patient care

---

content) at the beginning of the rotation so students know their future evaluation is based on shared learning objectives.

Ranking Performance

Many evaluations rank performance along a scale from poor to superior in relation to that of peers. This method is less useful than an assessment of performance in relation to the task objectives themselves. For instance, one useful rating scheme is "cannot comment/needs more observation/ needs improvement/effective/exceptional." Notations like these (taken from the Johns Hopkins General Internal Medicine Residency Program Community-Based Practice Evaluation Form) are more to the point of the teaching exercise: How well does the student perform the task you are measuring? Furthermore, the emphasis is on objectivity and personal observation.

Evaluative remarks should be specific and indicate precisely what needs more observation, what needs improvement, what the student does effectively, and so on. Preceptors should use the opportunity for summative evaluation to direct students in improving deficient performance. Where observation has been insufficient, they should be honest and devise a plan for adequate supervision of the particular skill in the future. This may need to be arranged through the program director for future rotations.

If possible, preceptors should comment on learners' progress toward their learning objectives. This input is especially valuable when they compare final achievement with that at midrotation or compare one rotation with the next over longer periods, since it helps students set learning goals for the future.

Direct Observation

Ideally, evaluations should be based on direct observation. Indeed, this is one of the great strengths of ambulatory teaching. Feedback is inherently more credible when teachers can tell students what they have seen. Too much advice on clinical performance is based on students' own reports of patient care, write-ups, or the observations of someone other than the preceptor (e.g., program director reporting on a summative evaluation). Furthermore, many competencies that students need to achieve (communication skills, history taking, physical exams) must be directly observed to be optimally evaluated. Setting aside an adequate number of visits during teaching sessions so that the teacher can watch the student in action improves the quality of feedback.

Clear, Specific Feedback

Feedback should be clear and specific. Clear comments with sufficient, relevant detail have the greatest influence on behavior. General comments such as "You're doing a nice job" are too vague. They may build rapport (and are fine occasionally), but they provide little useful information. Not only are students unable to identify exactly what aspect of the "job" they are doing nicely, but they may be led to overestimate their accomplishment. Perhaps the student takes the comment to mean he is a star, when in fact his work is satisfactory. One can only imagine his disappointment if, based on this misunderstanding, his final grade is good rather than great. Well-stated, maximally informative feedback identifies what the teacher wants the student to know. A statement such as "You put the patient at ease by introducing yourself and telling her what you planned to accomplish" is superior to simply saying, "You put the patient at ease."

Objective and Subjective Feedback Statements

Objective comments are preferable to subjective ones. Objective statements are nonjudgmental and simply state the facts as you see them. They have the merit of being relatively irrefutable and therefore not contentious. For instance, the teacher can state (at the proper time), "I see that you did not palpate the patient's heart before using your stethoscope. By failing to do this you miss the chance to feel the location and quality of the apical beat," thus leaving little room for dispute. Were the teacher to say, in a subjective vein, "You will never master the cardiac exam unless you palpate the heart before auscultation," the statement might be true, but it is inherently judgmental and more likely to engender an emotional rather than an intellectual reaction. Subjective comments may be motivational in the proper context; this admonition may motivate the student to master the heart exam. But subjective statements should be identified as personal bias ("In my opinion you will never master...") and used very carefully. It is not hard to see how they may discourage rather than encourage a student.

While it is ideal to give feedback immediately, this is not always possible or realistic. It may be inappropriate during an emergency, during or immediately after an emotionally trying patient visit, when it interferes with patient care, or after an embarrassing failure by the student. In any of these situations it is wiser to save corrective feedback for later when the student is likely to be receptive.

Starting Formal Evaluative Sessions

How feedback is delivered is obviously important. As I mentioned before, the student should be prepared to hear it, the amount should not be overwhelming, and it should be delivered in a supportive, problem-solving manner.

Formal evaluative sessions may be intimidating until students become accustomed to receiving feedback and trust that their preceptors are promoting their welfare. Because students are usually apprehensive about being judged, it is best to set an encouraging tone. A friendly expression and a reassuring greeting help. Feedback sessions should be scheduled to permit adequate time for discussion—neither the student nor the preceptor should feel rushed. It is also a good practice to begin formal feedback sessions by stating the purpose of the meeting and laying out the goals, using a collaborative format that allows the student adequate input. After outlining what she would like to accomplish, the preceptor can open a dialogue by posing a question such as, "How do you think the rotation has gone so far?" Most students are not reticent about sharing their feelings; they are usually quite willing to identify what works, what doesn't, and what would work better for them. If the student seems shy about making substantive comments, the preceptor should offer a few questions to get the conversation started. She can refer to the learning contract and ask, "Do you feel you are meeting the goals in our contract?" "What teaching activities are helping you meet your learning goals?" "What could I do better to help you reach these goals?"

Once the conversation is begun the teacher and student can concentrate on the specifics, based on the student's needs and the preceptor's understanding of the course objectives. During the discussion the preceptor should use informational and motivational feedback to address the student's strengths and weaknesses. At some point the preceptor should ask, "Do you feel you're receiving enough feedback?" The student and preceptor then develop specific plans for formative feedback sessions, and these points are summarized orally. Both parties adopt commitments and a plan for implementing change. The preceptor should also document the discussion for future reference.

Wording Feedback

When delivering feedback during formal and informal sessions, wording is important. In general feedback should be worded positively to encourage the student. Negative feedback, though it may be necessary too, should never be disparaging. When you have to deliver negative feedback, it will be more easily received if the student is confident and has good rapport with the teacher and if previous feedback has been sufficiently positive.

Sequencing positive and negative feedback is important as well. Negative feedback is more readily accepted if it is preceded by positive feedback or even sandwiched between positive statements. The usual technique is to make a relevant positive feedback statement followed by a relevant negative one.

A preceptor observes a medical student fishing around in a patient's bag of med-icines while he gives her instruction for taking a new drug. The preceptor wants the student to recognize that his distracting behavior interferes with the patient's concentrating on his instructions. To improve acceptance of the feedback, he praises the student's care in checking her prescription bottles, then notes how the distracting activity reduced the effectiveness of his communication. He says to the student, "You did the right thing by checking and recording all the patient's med-ications. However, by looking at the medication bottles while you were giving her instructions, you diminished her ability to concentrate on what you were telling her. The best practice is to perform patient education when you can look the per-son in the eye and give her your undivided attention."

On the other hand, this technique—the "good news before the bad"—has flaws. Irrelevant positive feedback that precedes negative feedback may appear disingenuous. For instance, forced positive feedback that serves no genuine purpose looks phony and reduces credibility. This would have been the case had the preceptor in the previous example be-gun, "I liked the fact that you asked the patient about her ability to afford the new prescription. However, by looking at her medications while..." The opening line has no obvious connection to a major point of instruc-tion. It looks like a blatant attempt at softening the correction.

Positive feedback may also diminish the impact of an important neg-ative message. For this reason it is sometimes preferable to let negative feedback stand alone, as when the preceptor wants to deliver a strongly worded message. If a student needs to be confronted about a serious be-havioral flaw, then sugarcoating blunts the negative message and makes it less effective.

A preceptor decides he must confront a student about habitual tardiness. He could begin by telling the student, "John, I really appreciate your help in the office, and I recognize that you stay until the work is done, but your habitual tardiness keeps patients waiting and the staff running overtime." This buffer, although well inten-tioned, trivializes the seriousness of the message. An honest, straightforward statement delivers it more effectively: "John, I must tell you that your habitual tardiness keeps patients waiting and the staff running overtime. You will need to be here at our agreed-on time."

When and how to deliver strongly worded statements depends on the preceptor's judgment and knowledge of the student's receptivity.

Corrective feedback does not always have to be worded negatively, however. Particularly early in the student-teacher relationship, when rapport is developing but not firmly established, the teacher should phrase corrective feedback positively (or at least gently).

A student enters the preceptor's office to consult about a difficult patient he has just examined. The student is obviously frustrated because the patient has spoken to him rudely, and he refers to the patient using derogatory language. The attending does not want to let the statement pass without remark, but he does not want to make the student defensive either. He softens his remark about the inappropriateness of using a derogatory term for the patient by empathizing with the student's frustration: "I get upset with this patient too. However, rather than letting off steam by calling him a name, I recommend telling him what behavior you find unacceptable. When I see him, I lay down rules for acceptable conversation. I find that using epithets for such patients interferes with my treating them humanely."

The message must also be consistent with the teacher's tone of voice, facial expression, and body language. Teachers may not be aware that they sound stern or angry when they do not intend to. Perhaps they are simply harried owing to work. The opposite can be true as well—if they intend to deliver a serious message while adopting an insouciant air, perhaps they are anxious about having to deliver a difficult message. In any case, teachers must monitor nonverbal communication and make sure it is consistent with their intent.

An intern presents a patient's history to his attending while the attending, attempting to listen, is hurriedly jotting notes in a chart. The attending feels pleased with the intern's workup and tells him so. The intern does not "hear" this message; rather, he feels that the attending is bored with his presentation.

Including Students in the Discussion

Feedback is more easily digested when students make a personal contribution to the evaluation. As I noted before, preceptors can encourage this by soliciting students' self-appraisal and incorporating it into a discussion. A useful way to begin feedback sessions is to ask students how they feel about their progress toward their goals. Questions such as "How do you feel about your skill in taking a pertinent sexual history?" allow them to estimate their performance and ease into a discussion about areas in which they are having difficulty. It also gives teachers insight into students' perception of their achievement. Is it realistic or not? Sometimes it is helpful to have them enumerate their strengths and weaknesses for a particular task or area of study. By listing strengths as well as weaknesses, they do not focus exclusively on failure, and the feedback exercise does not challenge self-esteem.

Finally, feedback is more easily accepted when it is offered with a solution. Noting a deficiency without providing a remedy may leave students feeling anxious. Teachers can offer solutions or students may develop their own.

During a midmonth feedback session, a preceptor discusses record keeping with a pediatric resident. An audit of the resident's office notes reveals that they do not document evaluation and management sufficiently to justify the coding levels she is marking. The preceptor tells her that it took him a while to learn this also. To help her achieve satisfactory competency, he asks her to take copies of the notes and schedule a half-hour session with the billing clerk to get specific instruction. The resident leaves the session relieved. She does not worry about how she will achieve this objective and feels good about the feedback.

Follow-up and Reinforcement

Once feedback is given, preceptors must provide an adequate mechanism for monitoring progress. Good performance must be sustained and reinforced. The teacher and student should use feedback sessions to reevaluate goals and progress. Once advice has been given the teacher will need to ensure that it is followed through and that new behaviors are continued. Systematic reminders before targeted clinical situations will have the greatest effect in maintaining the desirable behavior.

Reciprocal Feedback from Students

Teachers should give students ample opportunity to give them feedback about their teaching, as I suggested in discussing summative evaluation sessions. However, preceptors can also get regular feedback during the course of teaching. Since students may be reluctant to offer feedback without prompting, preceptors should ask for their opinions regarding the learning content and about whether the teaching is helping them meet their goals, the workload and pace are acceptable, communication is clear, and so forth. It is very important that this be done early on, too. It is surprising that students will sometimes seem quite satisfied with teaching, at least going by their expressions, yet late in the rotation complain that they did not have enough of one or another experience or lesson. Preceptors can reduce the chance of this by asking about teaching frequently in the beginning. They should reassure learners that because students have different needs, their questions are for one purpose: to help them help students. Useful questions include:

1. Are you seeing the right number of patients?
2. Are you seeing the right mix of patients?
3. Do you feel you are getting the right amount of supervision?
4. Are there topics you would like to cover in more detail?
5. Are you getting an adequate opportunity to practice [specific skills]?
6. Do you feel comfortable with what is expected of you?
7. Do you feel you are getting the right amount of autonomy?

8. Which teaching method—lectures or independent study—has been more helpful to you?

9. Is there something I can do differently that will enhance your learning?

10. Are you getting adequate feedback on your performance?

Summary

• In evaluation, preceptors analyze students' performance and then provide feedback to correct mistakes, motivate behavior, or reinforce good practice.

• Formative evaluations are typically informal and concurrent with teaching. The major purpose is to provide the learner with timely feedback.

• Summative evaluations are scheduled sessions in which the preceptor and student engage in a dialogue to review overall progress toward learning goals.

• The feedback source is usually the preceptor, but it includes patients and the student's self-appraisal. To be maximally effective, feedback should be trustworthy and credible. In addition, feedback from different sources should be consistent.

• Ideally, evaluative feedback is timely, objective, and specific. Feedback that is delayed, subjective, or general provides little direction for changing behavior or continuing good practice.

• Positive feedback is preferred over negative feedback and eases the way for necessary negative feedback. Positive feedback is an effective motivational tool and is too often missing from clinical instruction.

• A mechanism should be created for monitoring performance and reinforcing success. Reminders and positive feedback are the most effective means of ensuring that the learner continues desirable behaviors.

• In addition to giving feedback, preceptors should frequently and systematically seek feedback from students. They can do so by creating a collaborative learning environment and asking students to assess the learning content, how effectively the teaching is meeting their needs, and whether preceptors are providing useful feedback.

REFERENCES

Alguire, P. C., D. E. DeWitt, L. E. Pinsky, and G. S. Ferenchick. 2001. *Teaching in your office: A guide to instructing medical students and residents.* Philadelphia: American College of Physicians–American Society of Internal Medicine.

Anderson, R. C., and G. W. Faust. 1973. *Educational psychology: The science of instruction and learning.* New York: Dodd, Mead.

Ausbel, D. 1968. *Educational psychology: A cognitive view.* New York: Holt, Rhinehart.

Baldwin, L. M. 1997. Managing clinic time while precepting medical students. *Fam. Med.* 29 (1): 13.

Beckman, H. B., and R. M. Frankel. 1994. The use of videotape in internal medicine training. *J. Gen. Intern. Med.* 9:517–21.

Behrman, R. E. 1996. Some unchanging values of pediatric education during a time of changing technology and practice. *Pediatrics* 98 (6): 1249–54.

Bennett, J., and F. Plum. 1996. Medicine as a learned and humane profession. In *Cecil textbook of medicine,* 20th ed. Philadelphia: W. B. Saunders.

Benzie, D. 1999. Community physician bookshelf. *Fam. Med.* 31 (2): 84–86.

Bloom, B. S., ed. 1956. *Taxonomy of educational objectives.* Book 1: *Cognitive domain.* New York: McKay.

Borum, M. L. 1997. Medical residents' colorectal screening may be dependent on ambulatory care education. *Dig. Dis. Sci.* 42 (6): 1176–78.

Burke, W., R. B. Baron, M. Lemon, et al. 1995. Training generalist physicians: Structural elements of the curriculum. *J. Gen. Intern. Med.* 9 (4, suppl. 1): S23–30.

Covell, D. G., C. G. Uman, and P. R. Manning. 1985. Information needs in office practice: Are they being met? *Ann. Intern. Med.* 103:596–99.

Darkenwald, G. G., and S. B. Merriam. 1982. *Adult education: Foundations of practice.* New York: Harper and Row.

Devera-Sales, A., C. Paden, and D. C. Vinson. 1999. What do family medicine patients think about medical students' participation in their health care? *Acad. Med.* 74 (5): 550–52.

DeWitt, T. G. 1996. Faculty development for community practitioners. *Pediatrics* 98 (6): 1273–76.

DeWitt, T. G., R. L. Goldberg, and K. B. Roberts. 1993. Developing community faculty: Principles, practice, and evaluation. *Am. J. Dis. Child.* 147 (1): 49–53.

Duckworth, K. S., M. W. Kahn, and T. G. Gutheil. 1994. Roles, quandaries, and remedies: Teaching professional boundaries to medical students. *Harv. Rev. Psychiatry* 1 (5): 266–70.

Ericksen, S. C. 1985. *The essence of good teaching.* San Francisco: Jossey-Bass.

Falvo, D. 1980. Patient perception as a tool for evaluation and feedback. *J. Fam. Pract.* 10:471–74.

Ferenchick, G., D. Simpson, J. Blackman, et al. 1997. Strategies for efficient and effective teaching in the ambulatory care setting. *Acad. Med.* 72:277–80.

Foley, R. P., and J. Smilansky. 1980. *Teaching techniques: A handbook for health professionals.* New York: McGraw-Hill.

Frank, S. H., K. C. Stange, D. Langa, and M. Workings. 1997. Direct observation of community-based ambulatory encounters involving medical students. *JAMA* 278 (9): 712–16.

Fulkerson, P. K., and R. Wang-Cheng. 1997. Community-based faculty: Motivation and rewards. *Fam. Med.* 29 (2): 105–7.

Gillis, J. S. 1993. Effects of life stress and dysphoria on complex judgements. *Psychol. Rep.* 72 (3, part 2): 1355–63.

Gordon, T. 1977. *Leader effectiveness training, L.E.T.: The no-lose way to release the productive potential of people.* New York: Wyden Books.

Grayson, M. S., D. A. Newton, M. Klein, and T. Irons. 1999. Promoting institutional change to encourage primary care: Experiences at New York Medical College and East Carolina University School of Medicine. *Acad. Med.* 74 (1, suppl.): S9–15.

Gruppen, L. D. 1997. Implications of cognitive research for ambulatory care education. *Acad. Med.* 72:117–20.

Hageman, P. A. 1988. Ratings of clinical clerkship feedback by allied health faculty and students. *J. Allied Health,* May, 115–21.

Harrow, A. J. 1972. *A taxonomy of the psychomotor domain: A guide for the developing behavioral objectives.* New York: David McKay.

Heikes, L. G., and C. L. Gjerde. 1985. Office procedural skills in family medicine. *J. Med. Edu.* 60 (6): 444–53.

Hinz, C. F. 1966. Direct observation as a means of teaching and evaluating clinical skills. *J. Med. Edu.* 41:150–61.

Hunter, K. M., R. Charon, and J. L. Coulehan. 1995. The study of literature in medical education. *Acad. Med.* 70 (9): 787–94.

Irby, D. M. 1978. Clinical teacher effectiveness in medicine. *J. Med. Edu.* 53:808–15.

———. 1986. Clinical teaching and the clinical teacher. *J. Med. Edu.* 61 (9, part 2): 35–45.

Jacobson, E. W., W. L. Keough, B. E. Dalton, et al. 1998. A comparison of inpatient and outpatient experiences during an internal medicine clerkship. *Am. J. Med.* 104:159–62.

Jaffe, A., D. Friedman, and B. Ritchen. 1985. Preceptorships in family medicine for second-year medical students. *J. Med. Edu.* 60:197–200.

Jaffe, C. C., and P. J. Lynch. 1996. Educational challenges. *Radiol. Clin. North Am.* 34 (3): 629–46.

Kassirer, J. P., and R. I. Kopelman. 1991. *Learning clinical reasoning.* Baltimore: Williams and Wilkins.

Kearl, G. W., and A. G. Mainous. 1993. Physicians' productivity and teaching responsibilities. *Acad. Med.* 68 (2): 166–67.

Kern, D. E., P. A. Thomas, D. M. Howard, and E. B. Bass. 1998. *Curriculum development for medical education: A six-step approach.* Baltimore: Johns Hopkins University Press.

Kirz, H. L., and C. Larsen. 1986. Costs and benefits of medical student training to a health maintenance organization. *JAMA* 256 (6): 734–39.

Knowles, M. 1973. *The adult learner: A neglected species.* Houston: Gulf.

Kolb, D. A. 1976. *The learning style inventory: Technical manual.* Boston: McBer.

———. 1985. *Learning style inventory.* Boston: McBer.

Krathwohl, D. R., B. S. Bloom, and B. B. Masia. 1980. *Taxonomy of educational objectives.* Book 2: *Affective domain.* New York: Longman.

Langlois, J. P., and S. Thach. 2000. Teaching at the bedside. *Fam. Med.* 32 (8): 528–30.

Lavizzo-Mourey, R., L. H. Beck, D. Deserens, et al. 1990. Integrating residency training in geriatrics into existing outpatient curricula. *J. Gen. Intern. Med.* 5 (2): 126–31.

Lesky, L. G., and W. Y. Hershman. 1995. Practical approaches to a major educational challenge. *Arch. Intern. Med.* 155:897–904.

Lipsky, M. S., and M. Egan. 1999. Students as assets. *Fam. Med.* 31 (6): 387–88.

Lowry, M. 1997. Using learning contracts in clinical practice. *Prof. Nurse* 12 (4): 280–83.

Menahem, S., and P. Shvartzman. 1998. Is our appearance important to our patients? *Fam. Pract.* 15 (5): 391–97.

O'Malley, P. G., D. M. Omori, F. J. Landry, J. Jackson, and D. Kroenke. 1997. A prospective study to assess the effect of ambulatory teaching on patient satisfaction. *Acad. Med.* 72 (11): 1015–17.

Opila, D. A. 1997. The impact of feedback to medical housestaff on chart documentation and quality of care in the outpatient setting. *J. Gen. Intern. Med.* 12 (6): 352–56.

Osborn, L. M., J. R. Sargent, and S. D. Williams. 1993. Effects of time-in-clinic, clinic setting, and faculty supervision on the continuity of clinic experience. *Pediatrics* 91 (6): 1089–93.

Qualters, D. 1999. Observing students in a clinical setting. *Fam. Med.* 31 (7): 461–62.

Quattlebaum, T. G. 1996. Techniques for evaluation of residents and residency programs. *Pediatrics* 98 (6): 1277–83.

Roberts, K. B. 1996. Educational principles of community-based education. *Pediatrics* 98 (6): 1259–63.

Rubenstein, W., and Y. Talbot. 1992. *Medical teaching in ambulatory care: A practical guide.* New York: Springer.

Sachdeva, A. K. 1996. Use of effective feedback to facilitate adult learning. *J. Cancer Educ.* 11 (2): 106–18.

Schwenk, T. L., and N. A. Whitman. 1987. *The physician as teacher.* Baltimore: Williams and Wilkins.

Speedling, E. J., and D. N. Rose. 1985. Building an effective doctor-patient relationship: From patient satisfaction to patient participation. *Soc. Sci. Med.* 21 (2): 115–20.

Steele, D. J. 1997. Orienting medical students in community-based teaching sites. *Fam. Med.* 29 (9): 614–15.

Swick, H. M. 2000. Toward a normative definition of medical professionalism. *Acad. Med.* 75 (6): 612–16.

Tamblyn, R., S. Benaroya, L. Snell, et al. 1994. The feasibility and value of using patient satisfaction ratings to evaluate internal medicine residents. *J. Gen. Intern. Med.* 9:146–52.

Usatine, R. P., and K. Lin. 1998. Cool Web sites for community preceptors. *Fam. Med.* 30 (7): 475–76.

Usatine, R. P., P. T. Tremoulet, and D. Irby. 2000. Time-efficient preceptors in ambulatory care settings. *Acad. Med.* 75 (6): 639–42.

Vinson, D. C., and C. Paden. 1994. The effect of teaching medical students on private practitioners' workloads. *Acad. Med.* 69 (3): 237–38.

Vinson, D. C., C. Paden, A. Devera-Sales, et al. 1997. Teaching medical students in community-based practices: A national survey of generalist physicians. *J. Fam. Pract.* 45 (6): 487–94.

Weinholtz, D., and J. Edwards. 1992. *Teaching during rounds: A handbook for attending physicians and residents.* Baltimore: Johns Hopkins University Press.

Weitzman, M., L. C. Garfunkel, and S. Connaughton. 1996. Financing pediatric education in community settings. *Pediatrics* 98 (6): 1284–88.

Westberg, J., and H. Jason. 1993. *Collaborative clinical education: The foundation of effective health care.* New York: Springer.

Whitman, N., and M. K. Magill. 2000. The teaching moment. In *Precepting medical students in the office,* ed. P. M. Paulman, J. L. Susman, and C. A. Abboud. Baltimore: Johns Hopkins University Press.

Wright, S. M., D. E. Kern, K. Kolodner, D. Howard, and F. Brancati. 1998. Attributes of excellent attending-physician role models. *N. Eng. J. Med.* 339 (27): 1986–93.

Young, L. M. 1996. The perspective of the community pediatrician. *Pediatrics* 98 (6): 1255–58.